HUMAN SCIENCE OF DISASTER RECONSTRUCTION

An Interdisciplinary Approach To Holistic Health Following The Great East Japan Earthquake And Fukushima Nuclear Disaster

Waseda Institute of Medical Anthropology on Disaster Reconstruction (WIMA)

Project of Human Science of Disaster Reconstruction, Advanced Research Center for Human Sciences, Waseda University

Edited by Takuya TSUJIUCHI
Foreword by Richard F. MOLLICA

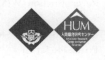

Human Science of Disaster Reconstruction
An interdisciplinary approach to holistic health following the Great East Japan Earthquake and
Fukushima nuclear disaster

Published by Interbooks Co., Ltd.
Kudan Crest Bldg 6F, 5-10, Kudan-Kita 1-Chome, Chiyoda-ku Tokyo 102-0073, Japan
URL: www.interbooks.co.jp/en/
Mail: books@interbooks.co.jp

Date of Publication
March 2019

Cover photo by Takuya TSUJIUCHI at Yuriage Minato Shrine, Miyagi Prefecture.
An enormous tsunami crashed over this hill, but the pine tree survived.
This shrine now watches over the many tsunami victims and
ensures the safe passage of their departed spirits.

©2019 Takuya TSUJIUCHI & Waseda Institute of Medical Anthropology on Disaster
Reconstruction (WIMA)

ISBN: 978-4-924914-61-2
Printed in Japan

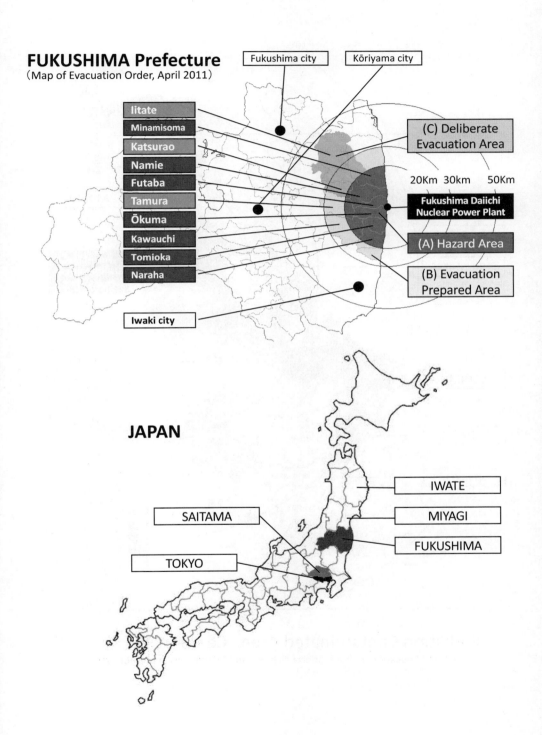

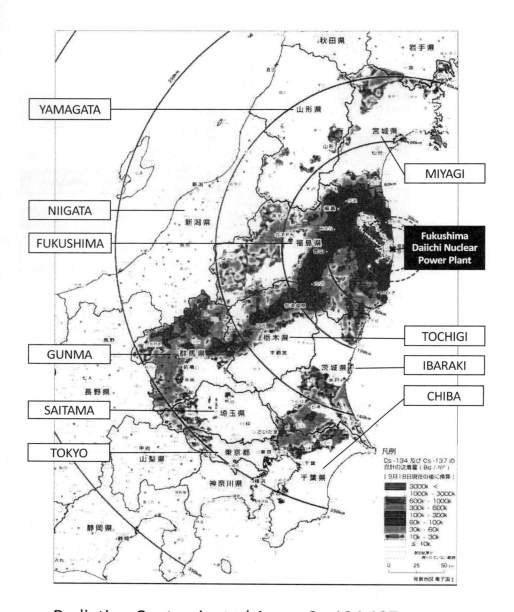

Radiation Contaminated Area, Ce-134,137
(Ministry of Education, Culture, Sports, Science and Technology, September 2011)

CONTENTS

CONTRIBUTOR'S PROFILE ix

FOREWORD
Lessons Learning from Great East Japan Earthquake and
Fukushima Nuclear Disaster
Richard F. Mollica, MD, MAR xix

INTRODUCTION
The Purpose of this Project
"Human Science of Disaster Reconstruction"
Takuya Tsujiuchi MD, PhD xxiii

**TOKYO GUIDELINES FOR TRAUMA AND
RECONSTRUCTION**
Formulating New Principles and Practices for
the Recovery of Post-Conflict Societies
Richard F. Mollica, MD, MAR, Yasushi Kikuchi, EdD xxvii

PART I
FIELD WORK & SUPPORTING ACTIONS

1 Mental Health / Community Health / Social well-being
The Emergency Evacuation Phase
—Fieldwork on nuclear accident evacuee support in Saitama
Takuya Tsujiuchi MD, PhD 3

2 Mental Health / Community Health / Social well-being
**How to Practice Social Care by Collaboration between
several professionality**
—Multi-vocal Analysis of Supporters
Jihye Kim CP, MA, Kazutaka Masuda CSW, PhD,
Takuya Tsujiuchi MD, PhD,
Shinsai Shien Network Saitama (SSN) 27

3 Physical Health / Public Health / Policy Making
Supporting the public healthcare system after a disaster
Tamotsu Nakasa MD,
Ryo Sasaki, Yasuo Sugiura, Yoichi Horikoshi, Jin Murakami,
Keiko Ouchi, Shinichiro Noda, Tomomi Kitamura,
Hidechika Akashi 55

4 Mental Health / Family Health / Community Health
Case study on support for voluntary evacuee families
—From records of social gatherings aimed at children
Ryuhei Mochida MA, Yuko Shiraishi MA 69

5 Physical Health / Community Health / Environmental Health
The Fukushima Support Project
—Development of radiological surveys to support
the building of safer environments
Hidetsugu Katsuragawa PhD, Taisuke Katsuragawa PhD 85

6 Community Health / Cultural Health / Human Security
Citizens Work Together to Overcome Disaster
Yuichi Sekiya PhD 97

PART II
RESEARCH PROJECT

1 Physical Health / Mental Health / Social Health
Mental Health Impact of the Great East Japan Earthquake
Eugene F. Augusterfer LCSW, Takuya Tsujiuchi MD, PhD 111

2 Mental Health / Community Health / Policy Making
Psycho-social Suffering and Structural Violence after the Fukushima Nuclear Disaster
Takuya Tsujiuchi MD, PhD 119

3 Mental Health / Public Health / Social well-being
Social Capital and Mental Health in a Major Disaster —Results of surveys and support after the Fukushima Daiichi nuclear power plant accident
Takahiro Iwagaki CSW, PSW, PhD, Takuya Tsujiuchi MD, PhD, Atsushi Ogihara PhD 145

4 Mental Health / Community Health / Social Well-being
Weakening Social Ties among Fukushima Evacuees and Providing Support
Kazutaka Masuda CSW, PhD 157

5 Mental Health / Community Health / Social Well-being
Relationships between psychological, social, and economic factors behind mental problems caused by experiencing disasters, and how to best provide social welfare support
Tsutomu Taga MA 169

6 Mental Health / Family Health / Community Health

Psychology of Families and Children Evacuated after Disaster

Koichi Negayama PhD, Shuzo Hirata MA,Konomi Ishijima MA,
Ryuhei Mochida MA, Yuko Shiraishi MA 181

7 Mental Health / Family Health / Community Health

How Evacuee Families with Children Adapt
—Considering relationships with their communities

Shuzo Hirata MA, Konomi Ishijima MA, Ryuhei Mochida MA,
Yuko Shiraishi MA, Koichi Negayama PhD 199

8 Mental Health / Community Health / Environmental Health

Analysis of living conditions and intentions of
out-of-prefecture evacuees fleeing the Fukushima nuclear
power plant accident

Noriko Ishikawa MA, Takaya Kojima PhD 217

9 Community Health / Policy Making / Social Security

Compensation for damages caused by the nuclear power
plant disaster

Hiroshi Kitamura 231

AFTERWORD

The Potential and the Future of Human Sciences
—Contributing to Disaster Recovery

Hiroaki Kumano MD, PhD 243

CONTRIBUTOR'S PROFILE

Takuya Tsujiuchi, MD, PhD

Professor, Faculty of Human Sciences, Waseda University
Director, Waseda Institute of Medical Anthropology on Disaster
Reconstruction (WIMA)

TAKUYA TSUJIUCHI M.D., Ph.D. is currently a professor at the Faculty of Human Sciences, Waseda University, and the director of Waseda Institute of Medical Anthropology on Disaster Reconstruction in Japan. After graduating from the School of Medicine, Hamamatsu University in 1992, he obtained his medical doctor license. He got a Ph.D. (Medicine) in 1999 at the Graduate School of Medicine, University of Tokyo where he specialized in stress sciences and psychosomatic medicine. After that, he entered another graduate school, the Division of Social Sciences and Humanities, Chiba University in order to study Cultural Anthropology. Since 2003, he has been lecturing in Medical Anthropology and Narrative Based Medicine in master and doctoral courses at Waseda University. He is also currently a lecturer of medical anthropology at the School of Medicine, Hamamatsu University and a board certified specialist physician at the Japanese Society of Psychosomatic Medicine.

During The Great Hanshin (Kobe) Earthquake of 1995, he worked as a volunteer medical doctor for the victims. His original paper, *Psychosomatic Problems after The Great Hanshin Earthquake in January 1995; Physical Stress Responses* (Jpn J Psychosom Med 36: 657-665, 1996) was given the 1997 Memorial Award by the Japanese Society of Psychosomatic Medicine. After the Great East Japan (Tohoku) Earthquake in 2011, Prof. Tsujiuchi has been supporting evacuees from the Fukushima nuclear disaster as a committee member of the private support group, Shinsai Shien Network Saitama (SSN), in the Saitama and Tokyo areas. He oversaw a research team and made a lot of quantitative and qualitative surveys to evaluate mental health and the social suffering of refugees from Fukushima. In 2013, he stayed in Boston, Massachusetts as a research fellow in the Harvard Program in Refugee Trauma (HPRT), Harvard Medical School, and Department of Psychiatry, Massachusetts General Hospital. In 2014, he established the Waseda Institute of Medical Anthropology on Disaster Reconstruction (WIMA) and started organizing holistic research to evaluate the medical (including mental health), socio-economic, and cultural issues that occur after disasters.

*Waseda Institute of Medical Anthropology on Disaster Reconstruction (WIMA)
URL: http://www.waseda.jp/prj-wima/
BLOG: http://blog.livedoor.jp/tsujiuchi_labo/

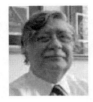
Richard F. Mollica, MD, MAR

Professor, Harvard Medical School
Director, Harvard Program in Refugee Trauma (HPRT)

Dr. Mollica is a professor of psychiatry at Harvard Medical School and director of the Harvard Program in Refugee Trauma (HPRT) at the Massachusetts General Hospital. Since 1981, Dr. Mollica and HPRT have pioneered the medical and mental health care of survivors of mass violence and torture in the U.S. and abroad. Under Dr. Mollica's direction, HPRT conducts clinical, training, policy, and research activities for populations affected by mass violence around the world. Dr. Mollica is currently active in clinical work, research, and the development of a global health curriculum, focusing on trauma and recovery. The Global Mental Health: Trauma and Recovery certificate program is the first of its kind in the field of global mental health and post conflict/disaster relief. Dr. Mollica has published over 160 scientific manuscripts and has recently published his first book, *Healing Invisible Wounds: Paths to Hope and Recovery in a Violent World* – Vanderbilt University Press, 2009.

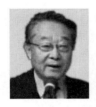
Yasushi Kikuchi, EdD

Professor Emeritus, Waseda University

Dr. Yasushi Kikuchi is a professor emeritus of Social and Development Anthropology at Waseda University, Tokyo. He received his Ed. D from De La Salle University. He is one of the pioneers in development anthropology and Philippine studies in Japan. He was visiting professor in Harvard University, Montreal University, Zurich University, De La Salle University, ESAN in Peru, and United Nations University. Since 1992, he is senior advisor to the Harvard Program in Refugee Trauma (HPRT) and has conducted several projects on the Kobe earthquake. He was appointed the presidential adviser to Peruvian president, Dr. Alejandro Toledo. The Peru Mental Health Program was initiated by him. He also established the Institute of Medical Anthropology at Waseda University in 2006. He was appointed policy adviser for international cooperation for the Foreign Minister of the Japanese Government from 2007 to 2009. Dr. Kikuchi has published several books and papers in various academic publications. The book *Human Relations and Social Developments* – New Day Publishers, 2014, covers all aspects of Dr. Kikuchi's long-term academic activities.

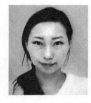

Jihye Kim, CP, MA

Graduate School of Education, University of Tokyo

Jihye Kim is a clinical-psychologist and research assistant at the Faculty of Human Sciences, Waseda University since 2015. She graduated in Human Sciences from Waseda university and got a master's degree in Clinical Psychology from Tokyo University. Now she is in a doctoral course for clinical-psychology at Tokyo University. Her research topics are psychological support for women and sexual minorities. As a clinical-psychologist, she provides guidance for psychological treatment and education for children with developmental disorders and supports psychological problems of adolescents.

Tamotsu Nakasa, MD

Visiting Professor, School of Tropical Medicine and Global Health, Nagasaki University

Tamotsu Nakasa currently serves as technical adviser to the Secretary General for Health, Republic Democratic of Congo and is a visiting professor at the School of Tropical Medicine and Global Health, Nagasaki University. For over 30 years, he has been conducting activities in the field of global health in Cambodia, Ethiopia, Bolivia, Pakistan, and Honduras. In the Great East Japan Earthquake of 2011 he also directed health support as an administrator at the National Medical Center for Global Health Medicine for Higashimatsushima City.

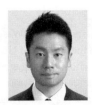

Ryuhei Mochida, MA

Visiting Researcher, Advanced Research Center for Human Sciences, Waseda University

Ryuhei Mochida is a fellow at the Advanced Research Center for Human Sciences of Waseda University in Saitama, Japan. After the Great East Japan Earthquake that occurred in 2011, he has investigated families who evacuated from Fukushima Prefecture to the Kanto region due to the damaged nuclear plant. His current research theme is about the loss of one's hometown and he has examined the grieving process and future prospects of evacuees. He obtained his master's degree in human sciences from Waseda University in 2012.

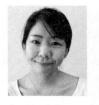

Yuko Shiraishi, MA

Research Fellow, Institute of Physical and Chemical Research

Yuko Shiraishi is a research fellow at the Center for Brain Science in the Institute of Physical and Chemical Research (RIKEN). She completed the doctoral program without a doctoral degree from the Graduate School of Human Sciences, Waseda University in 2017. Her current research interests are child development, child-parent relationships and parental support.

Hidetsugu Katsuragawa, PhD

Professor Emeritus, Toho University

Hidetsugu Katsuragawa is currently a professor emeritus at Toho University and visiting researcher at the Waseda Institute of Medical Anthropology on Disaster Reconstruction. He received a Ph.D. from the University of Tokyo in 1988. His research interest at Toho University was lasers-atomic nucleus physics. After retirement age, he was visiting professor at Toho University from 2007 to 2012. Since the Fukushima nuclear accident, he started volunteer work (Fukushima Support Project) with a group of scientists and engineers in May 2013. NHK featured TV programs that introduced activities of the Fukushima Support Project team several times.

Taisuke Katsuragawa, PhD

Associate Professor, Faculty of Human Sciences, Waseda University

Taisuke Katsuragawa (Ph.D. Human Sciences, Waseda University) is an associate professor in the Faculty of Human Sciences at Waseda University, Japan. He is a clinical psychologist engaged in educational counseling, developmental consultation, and supervision. He has written several books on children's clinical problems (e.g., bullying, school refusal, developmental disability) and published research papers on the counseling process. His current research interests cover the development of a measure for factors supporting children's autonomous development, the clinical significance of psychological examination in school education, and the predictability of clinical problems at school.

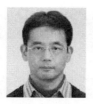

Yuichi Sekiya, PhD

Associate Professor, Graduate School of Arts and Sciences, University of Tokyo

Yuichi Sekiya is an associate professor of the Graduate School of Arts and Sciences, University of Tokyo. His specialties are cultural anthropology, development in Africa and disaster recovery issues in Japan. Soon, a book about public anthropology in the aftermath of disaster in Japan which he edited was published. (Yuichi SEKIYA and Hiroki TAKAKURA, ed. (2019) *The Public Anthropology of Recovery after the Triple Disaster in Japan: Collaboration with the Victims of the Earthquake, Tsunami, and Fukushima Nuclear Disaster*, University of Tokyo Press.) He obtained Ph.D. degree from the department of cultural anthropology in 2004 and worked for several institutes and colleges until his recent position from 2011.

Eugene F. Augusterfer, LCSW

Director of Telemedicine, Harvard Program in Refugee Trauma (HPRT)

Eugene F. Augusterfer is a senior faculty member and the director of telemedicine at the Harvard Program in Refugee Trauma (HPRT). As a clinician, he has been involved in clinical care for 30 years with a special interest in trauma informed care and post disaster recovery work. As director of telemedicine, he is responsible for planning, development and implementation of best practices, including teaching, supervision and mentoring of HPRT partners, to post-disaster areas. He has authored numerous published papers including *Telemental Health*, Elsevier 2012. He also co-edited and wrote a chapter in a book on *Telemental Health in Resource-Limited Global Settings*, Oxford University Press 2017. In addition, he is affiliated as a founding member of the Georgetown University Medical School – McLean Psychiatric Study Group and the World Bank Global Mental Health Working Group, and he did consulting for the World Economic Forum, Geneva, Switzerland on issues related to wellness. He served as a U.S. Air Force mental health officer and helped in the development and implementation of the USAF Telemedicine Program. After the Great East Japan Earthquake, he was invited as a key note lecturer by Waseda University, Japan, in 2013.

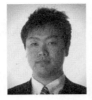
Takahiro Iwagaki, CSW, PSW, PhD

Visiting Researcher, Advanced Research Center for Human Sciences, Waseda University

Takahiro Iwagaki is a visiting researcher at the Advanced Research Center for Human Sciences at Waseda University. He received his Ph.D. in Human Sciences from Waseda University in 2017. Since 2015, he works as a staff member of the Area Comprehensive Support Center. He supports evacuees from the Great East Japan Earthquake of 2011. He carried out a large-scale questionnaire-based survey of evacuees from the Fukushima Daiichi Nuclear Power Plant disaster in collaboration with the Shinsai Shien Network Saitama (SSN). This survey revealed that losing one's local community by evacuation causes deterioration of mental health. He also revealed that trust and relationships with neighbors in everyday life are important for assistance in the event of a disaster.

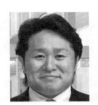
Atsushi Ogihara, PhD

Professor, Deputy Dean, Faculty of Human Sciences, Waseda University

Atsushi Ogihara is a professor and director of the Advanced Research Center for Human Sciences at Waseda University. His main areas of research are social medicine, social welfare, and regional vitalization studies. His Ph.D. in medicine is from Juntendo University. He obtained the United Nations University Akino Memorial Research Fellowship in 2004 and is a certified social worker and certified psychiatric social worker. He contributes to society as president of a non-profit organization for community social work. Dr. Ogihara also works as a member of the Health Planning Committee, Social Education Committee, and Policy Research Council in Tokorozawa City, Japan.

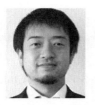

Kazutaka Masuda, CSW, PhD

Lecturer, Department of Psychology and Social Welfare, School of Letters, Mukogawa Women's University

Kazutaka Masuda is a lecturer in social work at Mukogawa Women's University, and editor of the *Japanese Journal of Home Care*. He is interested in advocacy with a focus on issues related to coordinated service delivery systems and access to care, particularly in the part played by front line implementers, and the creation of care management through different forms of knowledge. He has a practical background in voluntary sector community development work.

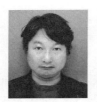

Tsutomu Taga, MA

Senior Researcher, Tokyo Metropolitan Institute of Gerontology

Tsutomu Taga is a researcher in the Research Team for Promoting Independence of the Elderly and Mental Health, Tokyo Metropolitan Institute of Gerontology (TMIG). He graduated with a B.A. in Biopsychology and a M.A. in social and clinical psychology from Keio University and with a M.A. in social welfare from Tokyo Metropolitan University. His research topics were social work practice, care manager's planning process, client and family caregiver's decision-making process on care planning, turnover problems of care workers, development of volunteer training programs, and prevalence of and living concerns regarding early onset dementia. He has been engaged in disaster reconstruction projects at Waseda University since 2015.

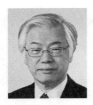

Koichi Negayama, PhD

Professor, Faculty of Human Sciences, Waseda University

Koichi Negayama is currently a professor of developmental human ethology in the Department of Human Environmental Sciences, Faculty of Human Sciences at Waseda University. He is a developmental psychologist with a Ph.D. from Osaka University. He served on the faculty at Osaka University from 1977 to 1986, at Mukogawa Women's University from 1986 to 1996, and at Waseda University from 1996 to present. His research interest is on the parent-offspring relationship in naturalistic settings. He was originally a primatologist working on mother-offspring aggression. His current research focuses on mother-offspring/inter-body relationships and negativity/parting (centrifugalism) with a special interest in feeding and weaning (kowakare), holding, and allomothering, etc.

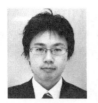

Shuzo Hirata, MA

Lecturer, Department of Child Studies, Sendai Seiyo Gakuin College

Shuzo Hirata is lecturer in the Department of Child Studies at Sendai Seiyo Gakuin College, and adjunct researcher at Waseda University. His specialties are developmental psychology and child welfare. The main focus of his research is life story work for foster children, which is one of the methods for supporting children whose memories are vague, unreliable, or inaccessible due to past experiences of separation or abuse. He has been working on the *Kasasagi* Project to survey and support families that evacuated to Kanto after the Tohoku Earthquake.

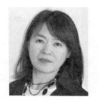

Noriko Ishikawa, MA

Graduate School of Human Sciences, Waseda University

Noriko Ishikawa is enrolled in the doctoral course at the Faculty of Human Sciences, Waseda University. Her field of research is architectural studies with a focus on architectural planning and environmental psychology. Currently, she is researching a residential-building-design support tool for eliciting the true and potential needs of customers, which they may not be conscious of. Since 1990, she has designed houses, clinics and apartment houses as an architect. She obtained her master's degree in human sciences from the graduate school of Waseda University.

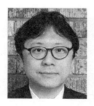

Takaya Kojima, PhD

Professor, Faculty of Human Sciences, Waseda University

Dr. Takaya Kojima is a professor in the Faculty of Human Sciences at Waseda University. His main field of research is architectural studies, especially architectural environmental studies and environmental psychology. He received his Eng.D. degree from the University of Tokyo in 1997. From 2000 to 2006, he was a senior researcher at the Building Reasearch Institue, an organ of the Ministry of Constructon that later became the Building Research Institute of the Incorporated Administrative Agency. He became an associate professor at Waseda University in 2007, and has been in the present post since 2017. As one of his main books, he has published *Covariance Structure Analysis (SEM) and Graphical Modeling Learning with Excel* in 2003 (revised in 2013).

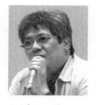
Hiroshi Kitamura

Senior Researcher, Institute of Politics and Economy

Hiroshi Kitamura is a political scientist. He is currently a senior researcher at the Institute of Politics and Economy, and a visiting researcher at Waseda Institute of Medical Anthropology on Disaster Reconstruction (WIMA). He was elected as an assembly member at Saitama prefecture from 2007 to 2011. Since 2011, as a deputy director of the private relief organization, Shinsai Shien Network Saitama (SSN), he participates in many projects supporting victims of the Great East Japan Earthquake and Fukushima nuclear accident. His research interests are philosophy of modern politics, contemporary social studies, and civil society movements. Recently, he has delved into several issues surrounding civil society, such us democratic principles and social exclusion and inclusion.

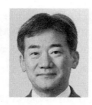
Hiroaki Kumano, MD, PhD

Professor, Faculty of Human Sciences, Waseda University

Hiroaki Kumano is a professor and former deputy dean of the Faculty of Human Sciences as well as former director of the Advanced Research Center for Human Sciences, Waseda University. He was trained at University of Tokyo (Ph.D. in Medical Science) and specialized in psychosomatic/behavioral medicine and is now educating university students on clinical psychology in medical settings. He has widely published in the fields of cognitive and behavioral therapies, relaxation and mindfulness, and the application of those fields for psychosomatic and psychiatric disorders.

ACKNOWLEDGEMENTS

The most important contributors to this project are the victims of the Great East Japan Earthquake and Fukushima nuclear disaster. All of the authors would like to express our sincere gratitude to all the victims reflected in our multiple surveys, the interview surveys, and the fieldwork studies. We admire the fortitude of the survivors as they conquered the numerous post-disaster difficulties.

We would like to also express our gratitude to Mr. Tadashi Inomata, Esq., the representative of the private support team "Shinsai-Shien Network Saitama (SSN)", executive officer Mr. Yutaka Aiko, Judicial Scriveners Mr. Takashi Hirose and Mr. Hiroyuki Nakagawa, clinical psychologist Ms. Yuko Hagiwara, clinical social worker Mr. Akihiro Takano, and all the members of SSN.

The authors also appreciate the valuable advice and supervision provided byProfessor Richard F. Mollica at Harvard Program in Refugee Trauma (HPRT), Dr. Tsunehiro Yasuda of Massachusetts General Hospital, Professor Yasushi Kikuchi, Professor Masao Nishimura, Dr Marisa Tsuchida, Dr. Fuyuki Makino, and Mr. Sumitoshi Sato. Also, without the contributions of all the co-researchers and many students of the graduate school of Human Sciences and Waseda Institute of Medical Anthropology on Disaster Reconstruction (WIMA), we could not have achieved these research findings.

Our publisher, Interbooks Co., Ltd, has been consistently helpful, patient and understanding in our endeavor. We wish to thank all the others who worked on this book, especially the translator who successfully took on the scientific English translation.

Finally, we wish to express our deep gratitude to all the encouragement, support and funding bestowed upon us by the Faculty of Human Sciences and Advanced Research Center for Human Sciences, Waseda University. A special thanks goes to Professor Hiroshi Fujimoto, dean of the Faculty of Human Sciences and Professor Akio Tanigawa, former dean of the same faculty.

FOREWORD

Lessons Learning from Great East Japan Earthquake and Fukushima Nuclear Disaster

Richard F. Mollica, MD, MAR[*1, *2, *3]

I am honored to have been invited to write a foreword to this pioneering and important volume by Japanese scientists and health care practitioners on the impact of the March 11, 2011 natural disaster in Japan known as the Great East Japan Earthquake. Violence from human and natural disasters is on the rise globally. Natural disasters are dramatically increasing and their impact on human life is vast; there are over 68 million displaced refugees worldwide and hundreds of millions of people displaced by climate change. While a large percentage of people have been impacted by natural disasters and the changing environment, human violence towards plants, animals, and the Earth itself is at an all-time high. Yet these researches in their science and through their humanity bring hope not only to survivors of the recent earthquake in Japan but to survivors all over the world.

When Professor Yasushi Kikuchi and I led the Waseda-Harvard mental health team in Kobe, Japan, amidst the broken city that was still on fire, we found courageous Japanese relief workers and citizen survivors working in a setting where disaster relief, mental health protocols, policies and intervention were in their infancy. As revealed in this volume, Japanese society and political leadership have been moving away from the stigma and ostracism associated with the emotional suffering secondary to traumatic life experiences. But, as is revealed, progress in Japan still needs to be made to have a comprehensive, holistic approach that restores the health and well-being to traumatized persons—maybe even policies that can foster post-traumatic growth.

---

*1 Director, Harvard Program in Refugee Trauma (HPRT), Massachusetts General Hospital
*2 Professor of Psychiatry, Harvard Medical School
*3 Honorary Advisor, Waseda Institute of Medical Anthropology on Disaster Reconstruction (WIMA)

In Kobe, I learned first-hand of the tremendous dignity and resiliency of the Japanese people and their culture. One of the most precious moments in my life occurred when I was in a shelter in a school interviewing earthquake survivors. Thousands were living together cramped into a small space. Each family's "home" was a small tatami mat. An elderly Japanese woman who had lost everything invited me to sit next to her and offered me some tea. We shared delightful tea and company for hours together as she told me about the disaster. This moving experience taught me a basic truth that I came to live by in medicine and life—that two people from radically different cultures can share together in an empathic and affectionate experience.

The researchers in this volume are emblematic of the great dignity, resourcefulness, and resiliency of the Japanese earthquake survivors. Disaster relief is primarily about restoring survivors to wellness, a sentiment which is echoed in this volume. I commend and offer gratitude to Professor Takuya Tsujiuchi and his colleagues for offering us this excellent volume.

INTRODUCTION AND TOKYO GUIDELINE

INTRODUCTION

The Purpose of this Project "Human Science of Disaster Reconstruction"

Takuya Tsujiuchi MD, PhD[*1, *2]

On March 11, 2011, the event known in Japanese as the Great East Japan Earthquake began. A catastrophic earthquake – magnitude 9.0 on the Richter scale – set off a massive tsunami that reached heights as high as 15 meters, and that, in turn, led to a crippling, Level 7 nuclear power plant accident. The unprecedented triple disaster resulted in the internal evacuation of around 300,000 people, the largest internal displacement of Japanese citizens since the Second World War. People fled for their lives, losing their homes, loved ones, and livelihoods. They were separated from the people closest to them, saw their hometowns destroyed, and were cut off from their own personal histories. The psycho-social suffering, the sheer trauma generated by such an experience is immeasurable.

The researchers affiliated with our project team aimed to respond to the multi-layered suffering these events caused by providing support through harnessing their diverse areas of expertise, including physical, social, and psychiatric medicines, clinical psychology, behavioral and health sciences, human ethology, social welfare science, sociology, cultural anthropology, environmental engineering, architectural science, political sciences, and law (Figure 1). Each of us asked ourselves what we could do and what was being asked of us, and there began our collaboration of individuals aiming to practice the Human Science in a broad meaning.

---

*1 Professor, Faculty of Human Sciences, Waseda University
*2 Director, Waseda Institute of Medical Anthropology on Disaster Reconstruction (WIMA)

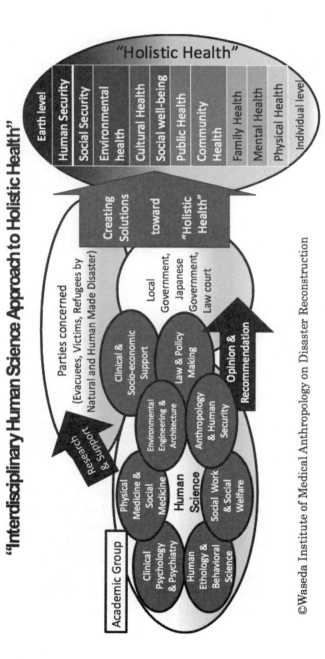

Figure 1. Mission of our project establishing interdisciplinary support action and researches.

The Human Sciences have always aimed to be interdisciplinary in nature, but they were in essence, as the plural term "sciences" suggests, a collection of different areas of expertise with different perspectives, all acting in parallel. There were difficulties in rising above that reality. However, the moment we obtained a shared objective – that of providing disaster relief in response to the 2011 Tohoku earthquake – a truly integrated academic discipline arose. It became a discipline in which experts shared a sense of mutual respect, a discipline in which they could overcome their different views and academic incompatibilities. That was the birth of the singular Human Science.

This book serves as a record of the social contributions required of academic activities during a large-scale disaster. The objective of our work was to provide holistic health care that spanned multiple levels, from individual to environmental, covering everything from physical, mental, family, community, and public health, to social well-being and healthy environments. At the beginning of each paper, the authors organize and present the three goals of their research, including how they connect to the above-mentioned levels of health care.

Part 1 provides reports on fieldwork and relief operations conducted by each researcher in the time immediately after the disaster. The activities described here have continued for the eight years since the earthquake and nuclear power plant accident.

Part 2 provides the results of the research projects. The fieldwork and relief operations described here are our response to the requirements of academic activities. The five papers by Iwagaki, Masuda, Taga, Ishikawa, and myself all describe the results of research conducted using the same survey data. The questionnaires used in the large-scale survey were created through a collaborative effort designed to get a comprehensive understanding of the issues faced by evacuees. Aiding in its design were many of the researchers involved in this project, supporters of the private relief organization Shinsai Shien Network Saitama (SSN), and even the victims of the disaster themselves. The deputy director of SSN, political scientist Hiroshi Kitamura, presented the complicated issues after the Fukushima disaster in the final article.

I serve as the lead researcher of this research project, which began with my work as a physician during the relief operations conducted after the 1995 Kobe earthquake. At the time, I was working in the Division of Psychosomatic Medicine at the University of Tokyo, and alongside the author of this book's afterword, Professor Hiroaki Kumano, I was writing a paper on the necessity of psychological health care in the practice of medicine. Similarly, at the time of the Kobe earthquake, Dr. Richard Mollica and Professor Yasushi Kikuchi, honorary advisors to this project, were pioneering efforts to successfully produce practical collaboration between the fields of disaster medicine and social anthropology. From 2013 to 2014, I had the opportunity to work under Dr. Mollica while a visiting research with the Harvard Program in Refugee Trauma (HPRT), and their trailblazing work left a great impression on me. I would like to open this book by presenting the Tokyo Guidelines for Trauma and Reconstruction, which these two individuals created almost 20 years ago. The subtitle of the guidelines, "Formulating new principles and practices for the recovery of post-conflict societies," hints at the comprehensive support required at different stages of the recovery process after a large-scale disaster. Even 20 years later, the guidelines seem just as valid in providing direct guidance towards finding a really important course to follow in the wake of such disasters.

The 21st century can surely be called the century of disaster. We face a future in which we can expect not only natural disasters including powerful earthquakes and destructive tsunamis, but also numerous human-induced disasters. Regarding nuclear power generation, there are more than 400 nuclear power plants in operation around the world and their numbers will increase in China and other emerging countries going forward. With these in mind, it is difficult to say that Chernobyl and Fukushima will be the last areas associated with the term "nuclear disaster." It must never be forgotten that major disasters result in extremely serious abuses of human rights. Ultimately, my hope is that the findings of this project, through the presentation of the idea of holistic health care, will contribute to the successful implementation of human recovery.

TOKYO GUIDELINES FOR TRAUMA AND RECONSTRUCTION

Formulating New Principles and Practices for the Recovery of Post-Conflict Societies

Richard F. Mollica, MD, MAR[1][2][4] *(Psychiatry, Global Mental Health),*
Yasushi Kikuchi, EdD[3][4] *(Social and Development Anthropology)*

Key words: Great Hanshin-Awaji (Kobe) earthquake, trauma,
reconstruction, development, policies

Introduction

The end of the twentieth century has seen an increase in societies devastated by mass violence. The world has also witnessed natural disasters of extraordinary proportions, such as the Great Hanshin-Awaji (Kobe) earthquake. Problems of violence and natural disaster and resulting trauma affect millions of people worldwide and will be central issues in the next century. Yet assistance in these "complex humanitarian emergencies" has remained largely unchanged or unchallenged since the end of World War II. One dilemma for international policy makers is that they do not have a scientific methodology for assessing the cultural, political, and social meanings of trauma in the lives of civilian populations and how these traumatic experiences alter the everyday lives of the affected individuals. Little empirical research assessing outcomes is conducted and humanitarian goals are often subordinated to political agendas. Although the magnitude of the problem is becoming clearer, methods for prevention and reconstruction of damaged societies have remained elusive. As a consequence, the enormous burden of human suffering and loss of social and economic productivity remains hidden behind a veil of neglect, ignorance, and denial.

---

[1] Director, Harvard Program in Refugee Trauma (HPRT), Massachusetts General Hospital
[2] Professor of Psychiatry, Harvard Medical School
[3] Professor Emeritus, Graduate School of Asian Pacific Studies, Waseda University
[4] Honorary Advisor, Waseda Institute of Medical Anthropology on Disaster Reconstruction (WIMA)

The Harvard Program in Refugee Trauma (HPRT) of the Harvard School of Public Health and Waseda University's newly created Institute for Asia-Pacific Studies (WIAP) recently received funding from the Japan Foundation Center for Global Partnership to organize a symposium addressing these issues. Taking place in May 1997 in Tokyo, this meeting brought together innovative thinkers to address the issues of economic and social recovery of communities extensively damaged by human and natural disaster. Equal time was given to the Bosnia-Herzegovina and Croatia, Cambodia, and Kobe, Japan. The participants gave brief lectures and participated in moderated discussions with the audience. The exchange of ideas exploring the political, cultural, and social meaning of trauma focused on the following themes:

-The impact of violence and natural disaster on personal, social, and community development;
-Scientific knowledge on the effect of mass violence and natural disaster on physical, psychosocial, and socioeconomic behavior;
-The role of the medical and mental health system in recovery and reconstruction of traumatized populations; and
-New policies for economic and social reconstruction of societies affected by mass violence and natural disaster.

The following conclusions and recommendations are the result of this exchange of ideas. A small working group drafted the guidelines and modified subsequent drafts based on the feedback from the symposium participants.

Tokyo Guidelines

1. Definitional Issues

1.1 The sequelae of trauma of individuals need to be defined and should include assessment of their health and mental health conditions, functional status, economic productivity and knowledge of the culture.

1.2 The impact of trauma on the ability of family, local community and, ultimately, national groups to affect the short-term and long-term recovery processes has been poorly defined.

1.3 Reconstruction should be redefined to include recognition that it is a complicated and broad- based process which requires more than simply repairing the infrastructure and restarting the economy of a country devastated by mass violence or natural disaster.

2. Ethical Decision Making

2.1 In the emergency phase to reconstruction continuum, field staff are often compelled to decide the "least worst" choice.

2.2 Organizations need to prepare their staff for ethical crises which arise because they are expected to remain neutral despite the fact that aid may be cynically manipulated by interested parties.

2.3 Organizations need to elucidate their ethical or moral "bottom line" for deciding whether to continue a relief or development operation.

2.4 Every professional and volunteer organization should clearly communicate standards of professional behavior to staff in ethical guidelines expressed through training and supervision.

2.5 Organizations should create institutionalized mechanisms for providers and recipients of relief services to engage in constructive dialogue and resolve conflicts.

3. Evaluation and Assessment Issues

3.1 For traumatic outcomes, a definition of "caseness" as a measurement of disability linking health and mental health to socioeconomic and sociocultural behavior has not been described.

3.2 Little analysis has occurred of the long-term impact of humanitarian assistance and development programs on traumatized populations.

3.3 Measurements have not been developed to assess the cultural efficacy of reconstruction activities. All recovery efforts should allocate resources to evaluate the cultural efficacy and socioeconomic success of implemented projects.

3.4 Funders and other interested parties should encourage organizations to scientifically evaluate their initiatives and try new approaches as well as abandon ineffective programs.

3.5 The potential benefit of media involvement in the relief to reconstruction continuum is still largely unknown and needs to be evaluated.

3.6 The relationships between tribunals and other reconciliation processes to reconstruction are unknown and need further study.

4. Emergency Phase to Reconstruction Continuum

4.1 The reconstruction process must be planned from the beginning of the emergency phase. In other words, recovery is nested within the earliest humanitarian response to trauma.

4.2 Knowledge about the natural history of the socioeconomic and sociocultural effects of trauma needs to be incorporated into planning for the emergency phase and subsequent humanitarian efforts.

4.3 Traumatized persons are often seen as powerless and needy and sometimes are forced into dependent situations which may have a negative long-term effect on their independent socioeconomic and sociocultural behavior. Standards of human dignity and human needs should be defined in a "gold standard" which planning organizations aspire to achieve in spite of limited resources and political agendas.

4.4 The emergency phase and subsequent reconstruction should be monitored by the implementers themselves in order to limit the possible and unintentional harm of humanitarian assistance.

5. The Importance of Altruism and Self-Help

5.1 Survivors of mass violence and natural disaster need to be given permission and empowered to do good by humanitarian and political authorities.

5.2 The international humanitarian assistance community needs more information about the capacities of traumatized populations to contribute to the reconstruction process. Scientific evidence clearly suggests that there is a surge of resourcefulness and mutual assistance early in the posttraumatic phase which can be utilized for recovery in spite of limited resources.

6. The Importance of Work

6.1 Trauma survivors will do whatever they need to survive. Although trauma survivors have been shown to maintain the ability to maximize survival in spite of high levels of psychosocial impairment, this productivity has rarely been harnessed in the recovery phase.

6.2 It is rare for individuals who have experienced traumatic events to limit their informal work activities (which we call "BIGS") despite conditions of extreme adversity.

6.3 In contrast, an individual's formal employment activity ("BEGS") is usually constrained by the existing sociopolitical environment and available economic opportunity.

6.4 Until jobs become available through formal employment, promotion of income generation through informal work activities is an essential foundation of the recovery process.

6.5 Small funds for self-recovery by survivors should be allocated during the emergency and long- term reconstruction phases.

6.6 There is a moral responsibility to take care of those who cannot care for themselves. Some people will be unable to participate in either formal or informal work activities even if they are provided with opportunities. These individuals need special assistance.

7. The Importance of Home

7.1 Planning for a permanent residence for survivors needs to be a top priority in the emergency phase.

7.2 Displaced populations need to be involved in the decision-making process with regard to choices and options related to housing. Local recipient communities, which are sometimes ignored during repatriation, need to be consulted as to the suitability of living conditions for newcomers.

7.3 Promotion of neighborliness is at the core of any long-term solution to difficult housing issues. Rebuilding neighborhoods and local community environments must replace concepts of repatriation and reconstruction which primarily focus on physical locations, structures, and transportation issues.

8. Vulnerable Groups

8.1 Vulnerable groups have a high burden of traumatic outcomes. Three vulnerable groups are of particular concern: Adolescents, the elderly and the mentally ill.

8.2 Since adolescents are often coping with despair about their future opportunities, addressing their special needs can help reduce their involvement in the cycle of violence.

8.3 The elderly are particularly burdened with solitary death, despair, and isolation.

8.4 In the emergency to reconstruction continuum, individuals seriously damaged psychiatrically by trauma and those with prior mental illness in the pre-trauma phase often have no access to mental health services; these services should be provided.

9. The Role of the Mental Health System in Reconstruction

9.1 Using scientific methods developed over the past twenty years, the health and mental health system can provide clinical care in a culturally sensitive way to traumatized populations and subgroups such as rape victims.

9.2 Mental health providers can serve as public health educators supporting local responses to the general community such as through the educational system.

9.3 Health and mental health professionals should participate in the process of reconciliation by maintaining a nonpolitical role and serving all affected populations regardless of ethnicity, social class, or political world view.

9.4 Recognizing the enormous stress on reconstruction organizations and their staff, technical assistance and training can be provided to reduce "burn out."

Bibliography

Colletta, N.J., Cullen, M., 2000. Violent Conflict and the Transformation of Social Capital: Lessons from Cambodia, Rwanda, Guatemala, and Somalia. Washington, DC: The World Bank.

Desjarlais, R., Eisenberg, L., Good, B., Kleinman, A., 1995. World Mental Health: Problems and Priorities in Low-income Countries. New York and Oxford: Oxford University Press.

Holtzman, S.E., Collin, A., 1998. Post-Conflict Reconstruction: The Role of the World Bank. Washington, DC: The World Bank.

Leaning, J., Chen, L., Briggs, S., 1999. Humanitarian Crisis: Medical and Public Health Response. Cambridge: Harvard University Press.

Mollica, R.F., 2000. McInnes, K., Sarajlic, N., Lavelle, J., Sarajlic, I., Massagli, M.P., 1999. Disability associated with psychiatric comorbidity and health status in Bosnian refugees living in Croatia. *JAMA*, 282, 433-439.

Mollica, R.F., 2000. Invisible wounds: Medical researchers have recently begun to address the mental health effects of war on civilians. *Scientific American*, 282, 54-57.

Murray, C.J.L., Lopez, A. (Ed.), 1996. The Global Burden of Disease: A Comprehensive Assessment of Mortality and Disability from Diseases, Injuries and Risk Factors in 1990 and Projected to 2020. Cambridge: Harvard University Press.

Part I

FIELD WORK & SUPPORTING ACTIONS

1 Mental Health / Community Health / Social well-being

The Emergency Evacuation Phase
Fieldwork on nuclear accident evacuee support in Saitama

Takuya Tsujiuchi MD, PhD[1, 2] (Medical Anthropology)

Key words: refugee, emergency support, social care, medical anthropology, Fukushima nuclear disaster

I. Going into the field

■ **11 April (Monday)**
Just one month has passed since the Tohoku Earthquake. I have few memories of anything that happened in the month. I do wonder exactly what I was up to in that time. I remember clearly that my wife was stranded in the city on the day of the earthquake, so I had to pick her up in the car and we got home the next morning. Then, from the explosion at the nuclear power plant, the radioactive material being found in the water supply, sending our kids to stay with their grandparents, food and water shortages, and the darkness of the repeated scheduled blackout, I think all that put me in a daze, and I ended up depressed. East Japan had been devastated, and I was buried in worry about the future of Japan, a future that had become so unclear.

Two or three weeks after the disaster, the news started showing the many people who had been saved from the damage caused by the tsunami, cheerfully talking about their aim for the rebuilding. Little damage had been done to Tokyo, and I started asking myself "What am I doing?" Compared to the people of Tohoku, I was not in a difficult position. I was pathetic. I knew that I had to find a way to restore myself emotionally. I somehow tried to lift myself out of the dark place I had found myself in.

---

*1 Professor, Faculty of Human Sciences, Waseda University
*2 Director, Waseda Institute of Medical Anthropology on Disaster Reconstruction (WIMA)

4   Part I - 1

An article in the newspaper on 1 April described how the entire population of Futaba – the town where Fukushima Daiichi Nuclear Power Plant is located – had been evacuated to Saitama Prefecture. The article said that approximately 2,000 people were living in at the closed-down Kisai High School, a former high school in the city of Kazo. I lived in Saitama as well, so I began thinking about what I could do to help.

Around 20 years ago, in February 1995, I was stricken by worry at images of the city of Kobe, devastated by a massive earthquake and subsequent fire, and the increasing numbers of dead being announced on the news. My father is from the Osaka/Kobe area. I was in my third year as a doctor, and I could to some extent handle basic emergency treatments and psychosomatic medicine. Maybe I could do something. Previously, after thinking about possibly working in overseas medical relief, I had become a member of the Services for the Health in Asian & African Regions (SHARE), a nongovernment organization that promotes health through international cooperation. Maybe SHARE would be sending doctors to the disaster area, I thought, so I quickly called the offices and told then I wanted to go to the disaster area, and they put me on the dispatch list. Just a few days later a fax arrived telling me the date I would leave. Memories of the Kobe Earthquake appeared in my head like flashbacks, and I decided to go to Kazo. Whatever I did, I had to go.

It was decided that I and other members of my laboratory would go to Kazo, Saitama – it was like my past self was at my back, and as if I was trying to inspire my present self. The team consisted of four members, including my research collaborator Katsumi Suzuki who I have been engaged in researching the "narratives of illness" for many years, and doctoral and master's degree candidates from the graduate school. As a university laboratory, we were looking for a sustainable way to offer our help for many years. For the previous decade, our research has involved listening to the stories of people with chronic and incurable illnesses and those dealing with disabilities and those facing death, then recording their words, and learning the wisdom these individuals had gathered throughout their lives. The other members of the laboratory were strongly in favor of going to Kazo.

We met on platform 3 at Ikebukuro Station, near the front car of the Shonan Shinjuku Line train leaving Ikebukuro at 11:15 for Utsunomiya. I bought some *ningyo-yaki* (Japanese traditional sweet) as a gift for the mayor of Futaba, Katsutaka Idogawa in case we got the chance to meet, and boarded the train.

What could we do? What sort of commitment could we make on site? Neither of these questions could be answered until we arrived and saw what we were dealing with. Our objective is to create interview surveys and ethnographies through long-term participant observation from the perspective of our own specialty, medical anthropology. However, research must not be done for research's sake. It has no meaning if it doesn't take a form that helps victims. As has been repeatedly witnessed in anthropological research, scientists must not exploit the lives and narratives of people living in the differing cultures of developing countries with the vocabulary of Western culture. I always try to follow that rule in my research into narratives of illness as well. As a former doctor of internal medicine and psychosomatic medicine, this was a research policy I had to maintain. Perhaps a means of providing mental health support as volunteers at first would be appropriate, but that decision would also have to wait until we saw the situation with our own eyes. Perhaps there would be something we could do as a university research institution rather than as doctors. It would also be possible to plan out questionnaires to get a better understanding of evacuee condition, and undertake quantitative data analysis, interviews regarding resident needs, and narrative analysis.

At 11:55, we arrived at Kuki Station. There we had to transfer to a Tobu Isesaki Line train bound for Tatebayashi, and we had about 30 minutes before our next train. We might be unable to get anything to eat once we reached our destination, so we filled up on warm sandwiches and coffee at the Starbucks in the station.

We arrived at Kazo Station at around 12:40. On a wall near the station gates were hung three *koinobori* in black, red and blue. A sign read "Welcome to Kazo – The *Koinobori* Town!" I remember that only a few days before, the news had reported that the city of Kazo had donated a whole set of *koinobori* to the evacuees from Futaba.

Kisai Saitama Prefectural High School – where the evacuees from Futaba, Fukushima were living – was located on a road about 4.2 kilometers south of Kazo Station. It wasn't too far to walk, but it was still pretty far. Kazo City Hall was only about one kilometer from the station. First, we decided to go to Kazo City Hall, which had accepted 1,200 evacuees from Futaba and allowed Futaba's town office to function there, and gather information by confirming conditions in the evacuation center and the support system.

II. Kazo City Hall Saitama Prefecture

Young green leaves clad the cherry blossom trees in full bloom beside the roundabout in front of the station. Above the trees, a large example of Kazo's famous *koinobori* was blowing in the spring wind (Figure1). I could feel a kind of power in it as it swam through the cloudy sky.

Kazo is located on the northern edge of Saitama prefecture, and is bordered by Ibaraki, Tochigi, and Gunma prefectures. It is famous throughout Japan for its traditional hand-painted koinobori, and during the Peace Festival held in Kazo every May, an enormous 100-meter-long *koinobori* is flown sky-high from a crane at a park beside the Tone River.

We left Kazo Station's north exit for our about one kilometer walk along a straight city road. Four and five story buildings lined the streets of the Ekidori Shotengai, a shopping district that stretches along the road from the station. The streetlights were covered in stained glass decoration, and there were also hanging flags decorated with a pair of cute koi fish and the words, "Welcome to Kazo." At the intersection near the entrance to Kazo City Hall, there were signs advertising dolls and koi, and an around three-meter tall sign that read, "Declared Human Rights City, Declared Health and Sports Promotion City, and Declared Nuclear-free Peace City."

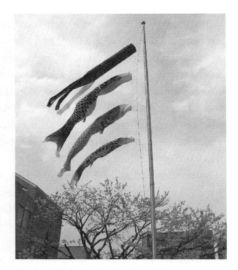

Figure 1. Koinobori and cherry blossom trees at Kazo

There were around thirty to forty cherry blossom trees around City Hall, a sturdy, five-story building clad in gray tiles. The city seemed to be in an economically sound position.

Just inside the entrance to the building was a pair of folding tables which were serving as a temporary consultation desk for questions related to the disaster. One male and two female employees were taking questions.

The Kazo City Futaba Town Relief Headquarters was run by the mayor of Kazo, and was comprised of nine sections: Public Relations, Volunteering, Environment, Employment Support, Welfare, Medical Care, Education, Food Relief, and a local contact office. The Policy Coordination Office of the General Policy Department had a volunteer section, and we were able to speak to its head, Mr. Takeyama (a pseudonym).

"There are currently 1,400 residents who evacuated from Futaba living at Kisai Saitama Prefectural High School. The school has been out of use for a while, so we had to reconnect the electricity, water, and gas to make it inhabitable, but it's already close to capacity. The toilet and sewage are at their maximum, as are the electric breakers," he said.

The biggest issue at this point is apparently that food cannot be prepared at the school because of some hygiene problems. All three meals each day continue to be comprised of *bento* (Japanese lunch) boxes or bread. They have a single rotary kettle that they can use to make miso soup. Apparently, once the children began going to school, parents wanted to be able to give them some miso soup before they left in the morning. Now, they cut up the ingredients elsewhere, and use them to make miso soup in the morning for breakfast. There are plans in place to bring a company in to clean the home economics classroom and see if it can be used for cooking. There are approximately 30 individuals in each classroom, and 80 people each in the judo hall, kendo hall, and gymnasium, so there are hygiene and privacy issues. Influenza is also prevalent, and it seems that one room is being used as an isolation room for people to recuperate.

"In terms of relief, the living volunteers are doing a lot. We announced this on the city's website as well, but we have temporarily stopped accepting new individual and group volunteers on April 3rd. We currently have 30 to 40 volunteers, bringing in supplies, carrying garbage, and distributing bento boxes, hot water, etc."

We were told that they still needed volunteers with special qualifications such as clinical psychologists, nursing care workers, and physical therapists. As a doctor of psychosomatic medicine, I was eligible to register as a volunteer, so I asked to have my name added to the registry.

Next, we met up with the head of the Health Care Department, Mr. Yamamoto (a pseudonym) so we could confirm the current state of medical relief.

"Saitama's Kazo Health Center has arranged to have a psychiatrist from Saitama Psychiatric Medical Center visit Kisai High School twice a week. It is necessary for people to receive mental health care during this period because they have started to worry about their future. When hospitalization and other sustained psychological care is deemed necessary, we have people looked at by Fudogaoka Hospital in Kazo. There are about 550 people with chronic illnesses living at the evacuation center. A medical practitioner from Futaba who evacuated with the other residents of the town is going to move to Tokyo, so the doctors from Kazo Medical Association who visit every week will be taking over. Doctors from Fukushima Medical University's Kanto Office also visit every Sunday to provide medical checkups, so I think our medical relief system is basically fully in place. We also have psychological counselling rooms set up, but I think many people probably find it difficult to visit those. The Saitama Bar Association has been offering legal and life counselling, but I've heard that most people who are coming are suffering from health problems."

Mr. Yamamoto apparently didn't think that the evacuation would end in one or two years. He also said that he would like to provide long-term support, and we saw that the city itself was taking a positive position on this. We were able to get a general idea of the support system, so our next stop would be to visit the people of Futaba living at Kisai High School.

III. Kisai High School Evacuation Center

We boarded the "Asahi Bus" leaving Kazo Station's north exit at 14:25 bound for Konosu Station and the Driver's License Center. The route offers around two buses an hour. We were on the bus for ten or fifteen minutes before we got off at Kisai-itchome bus stop.

The sky was dark with the sudden arrival of rain clouds, and a strong wind was blowing as rain began to fall. The frigid wind hit the back of our necks, chilling us to the bone. We walked a few dozen meters south of the bus stop and came out on National Highway 122. It was a broad, four-lane road, and it was mostly full of transport trucks. We walked northwest for another ten or so minutes. Among a sea of rice paddies in soil color, we saw the words, "*Gambarō* (Don't Give up) Tohoku! *Gambarō* (Do your best) Nippon!" We had arrived at Kisai Saitama Prefectural High School (Figure 2, 3).

The school grounds were packed with parked passenger cars, and there were ruts in the soil from their tires. In front of the school building was a mid-sized bus with the words "Futaba Town" written on it, and there were four or five TV trucks with their

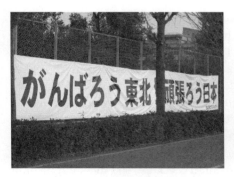
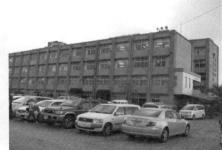

Figure 2. "*Gambarō* Tohoku, *Gambarō* Nippon"   Figure 3. Evacuation center at Kisai High School

The Emergency Evacuation Phase   9

parabolic antennas. There were two television crews carrying large video cameras on their shoulders, carrying stereo boom mics, or holding reflector panels, actively interviewing residents. A sense of starkness seemed to hover over the disordered, restless atmosphere.

A sign near the entrance to the school building read, "Volunteer registration has ended. Thank you for your cooperation. Kazo City Hall." The office was located on the second floor at the top of a flight of outdoor stairs, and there was a poster on the glass door that read, "Members of the media are not permitted past this point." We entered the building to find a square entry hall three meters wide, and a jumble of 20 to 30 pairs of shoes on the floor. We each took slippers out of cardboard boxes, and moved towards the temporary reception table in the hall.

There was an employee with a name tag hanging from the shoulder on a blue string and wearing a light blue work jacket. He looked up with a smile and greeted us with a "Hello". Apparently, he was an employee of Kazo city working in support of the evacuation center at Kisai High School. He seemed to be there to greet a lot of visitors with a smile, and to keep suspicious individuals out. I introduced myself.

"Hello, my name is Tsujiuchi and I am from Waseda University. A short while ago I met up with the heads of the volunteer section and medical care section at Kazo City Hall, and I have been registered as a volunteer doctor. I'm here today to see if I could speak to the mayor, if he has a moment."

The secretary in the Futaba mayor's office told us that the mayor was in a meeting and then she asked us if we could wait on the long benches in the hallway for a while. The floor of the hallway was gritty with dust, and it felt like there were echoes throughout the air.

A poster for Hello Work could be seen beside the room diagonally across the hall from the bench. It seemed to be a work placement program for evacuee residents. A woman around 30 angrily came out of the room, snapping the words, "There's no use coming here!" We could sense how important but difficult it was for the residents to find a job.

"Please come in," we heard the secretary say, so we opened the door to the mayor's office. It was once used as the school principal's office, but it is now being used as the mayor's office. The floor was covered with a plain grey carpet, and in the middle of the room was a worn, wooden meeting table and six pipe chairs with arm rests. There was a wide, wooden desk by the window that perhaps was once used by the principal. On either side were thousand *origami* paper cranes and numerous pieces of colored square message cards from supporters of Futaba. Above them, there was still a wall panel that had the words of Kisai Prefectural High School's school song written on it. On the wall next to the hallway was a small sink, and the shelves were piled with clippings from recent newspapers. Maybe it was the mayor who clipped all those out. We could still sense the bustle of the evacuation center, but there was an air of calm in the drab room.

I handed the mayor our gift of *ningyo-yaki* and spoke about how we were visiting to see if there was a way for us to engage in survey research and help the town rebuild as a university in the same prefecture. Mayor Katsutaka Idogawa is a short, quiet man. The hardships he has already faced are visible in his pure white hair and wrinkled forehead. His face told the tale of a powerful fatigue, but he listened sincerely to us the entire time, nodding as we spoke. When we were done, he waited a moment before beginning to speak softly in a hoarse voice that seemed to come from deep in his chest.

"There are some incredibly wide gaps that suddenly opened up in front of us," Mayor Idogawa said. "The unreal has become real. The gaps are awful. A gap in the environment, a gap in location. However, there is no way to measure how much the residents of the town feel those gaps. Perhaps if you could study that, you might find some interesting data."

I got a sense of his intelligence after he correctly assessed our intentions for our survey and research and proposing a research topic for us to attempt. Generally, people feel as if they should refuse when confronted with the possibility of surveys or research. However, Mayor Idogawa could look upon real phenomena at a higher level, from the broader perspective of history, therefore was able to intuitively understand the necessity for research and study.

"In a sense, bringing the residents of Futaba to Saitama is a pilot study as well," Mayor Idogawa said.

Pilot study is a term used in the social sciences to describe a study limited to a certain place and period, carried out to determine effectiveness and uncover potential problems before the introduction of a new system or technology. Another important element of pilot studies is the opportunity to exchange opinions with local residents, inform the public, and build consensus.

"Japanese society is made up of laws built upon laws, and it is becoming a society in which it is impossible to do what is needed," the mayor said. "And that has begun to make me feel unescapably trapped. I met the Minister for Internal Affairs recently, and he said that we are in a situation with no precedent, which makes it difficult to move things forward based on current legislation. He thinks we need to act based on extra-judicial thinking. I think these events give us a good opportunity to break free of this situation."

I was deeply impressed by his excellent sense of judgement as a mayor, even when faced with such a dreadfully extreme situation. He reminded of the figure of a native North American chief, standing up against the tyranny of the US government and its theft of the native people's land and resources. In a good way, the mayor in front of us was like the chief of an ethnic minority tribe.

"I think these events have brought us to a crossroads in how we solve our energy problems. Is nuclear power okay? How do we find alternative sources of energy? With the limited resources available on our planet, how do we get energy? I think we have to take this as an opportunity to discuss these questions. We cannot simply allow decisions to be made based on the opinions of people in positions of authority. This is a discussion we must all take part in," Mayor Idogawa continued.

The town of Futaba has lived side-by-side with the nuclear power plant for 50 years, and in that time has overcome various situations. Originally, farms could be found scattered across the region, and it is said that many of the residents were either engaged in farming or maintained homes in Futaba as they worked in Tokyo. In 1960, it became a candidate location for the nuclear power plants promoted by the national government, and Futaba and the adjacent town of Ōkuma accepted the plan. Construction of the nuclear power plant began in 1967, and the plant began operating in 1971. Many residents later began to work for the plant and other related companies, and the area received national grants earmarked for promoting areas with power plants. Moreover, corporate taxes paid by the power plant and other related companies began to pour into town coffers, and for a time, the town profited greatly. However, over-investment in public works projects and other issues caused Futaba to go into major debt in the early 1990s. The town council unanimously adopted a resolution to expand the nuclear plant, and the town began receiving new subsidies from the national government in 2007. Then, under Mayor Idogawa, the town had managed to rebuild its finances by 2009. This was the calm before the storm.

Regardless of any approval or disapproval toward nuclear power, the residents had no choice but to accept the nuclear power plant built in accordance with national and local government policies, and before they knew it, they had come to believe in the myth of the plant's safety and accepted the economic benefits it brought. Then came the triple disaster – the earthquake, tsunami, and nuclear accident – and they were forced to abandon their homes and drift through their country as each an internally displaced persons (IDPs). What have these people thought and felt over the last 50 years? I thought that there would be great value in recording each person's irreplaceable experiences for future generations to learn from. "I think you are right," Mayor Idogawa responded. "What is important is not just to record history, but to do so in a way that it can be easily passed on for later generations to use. This event can be used as a teacher or a textbook, a resource for people considering future development. I think this must be done."

We discovered that the mayor shares some of our intentions, and it seemed likely that we would be able to cooperate in the future. We made an appointment for our next meeting and left the mayor's office.

IV. Research survey proposal

■ **21 April (Thursday)**
We looked over the Waseda University Earthquake Recovery Project proposal that we would present to the mayor and had worked on until late the previous night. Which of these ideas would Mayor Idogawa be interested in? We had prepared five proposals for research that would be useful to Futaba now and in the future.

1. Get involved in community rebuilding
2. Conduct interviews regarding the hardships of life for residents
3. Generate a local history/record narratives
4. Make a record of the mayor's activity
5. Create a set of standards for third-party evaluations of reconstruction

When we arrived at the Futaba evacuation center at Kisai High School, the secretary told us that the mayor had been called away to deal with an urgent issue, but that the deputy mayor would be receiving us. The town of Futaba must have had to constantly deal with emergencies, and it must have been overwhelming to deal with these events as they occurred one after another. As we waited, an announcement was made throughout the school.

"Please note that the buses taking elementary and junior high students to the baths will depart at 4 PM and 4:40 PM. Please make sure to bring your bathing items, and gather at the bus stop. We also announce that non-students can take advantage of buses leaving at the same time for bathing facilities for the general public."

It seemed that they were now able to offer priority to evacuees in elementary and junior high school. Many elementary students stood in front of the entrance with

The Emergency Evacuation Phase   13

backpacks on their backs and chatting happily with each other. For each of them, the tatami mat spaces in the classrooms had become their family homes. How did these children feel about living in these conditions? We waited about 30 minutes, then were shown in to meet Deputy Mayor Kazuyoshi Inoue.

"I am very sorry for making you wait, and I apologize that the mayor cannot be here for your appointment," he said.

"It's no problem whatsoever," I answered. "I'm sure the emergencies are never-ending. It's a pleasure to meet you. My name is Tsujiuchi, and I work for Waseda University. I originally worked as a clinical physician in internal and psychosomatic medicine, but for the last ten years, I have specialized in medical anthropology, and have been researching health, welfare, and community issues from a broader social and cultural perspective. We visited the mayor ten days ago to ask if there was anything we as a university research institute could do to help, and we spoke to Mayor Idogawa for around 30 minutes. Mayor Idogawa responded favorably and allowed us to make an appointment with him for today to discuss our next steps in a more concrete way."

"I see," the deputy mayor answered. "In that case, can I assume that this is not your first experience dealing with such a situation?"

"Yes, I was a volunteer doctor providing medical examinations after the Kobe Earthquake in 1995, and I studied physical and mental issues that people faced. My recent work is explained in the documents we prepared. As a part of a collaborative regional work project in Tokorozawa city, I conducted interviews and questionnaire-based surveys designed to clarify the living situation for residents of working age and the health policies for small and medium-sized enterprises in the city. Then I provided recommendations at city meetings on health policies that would become necessary in the future."

In addition to our project proposal documents, we also brought with us a pamphlet from the Faculty of Human Sciences at Waseda University and a report from the collaborative regional work project in Tokorozawa, in order to provide a picture of who we were and to build a strong, trusting relationship.

"We would like to carry out our project after hearing your ideas and those of the mayor, so we can get an idea of what Futaba needs," I said. "We have no desire to do anything unilaterally, and we aren't looking at being temporary volunteers. Our intention is to continue for five to ten years and keep a close relationship with everyone even after they are able to return to Fukushima."

Deputy Mayor Inoue told us about the difficult conditions the residents of the evacuation center were in.

"It's already been a month since the disaster, but people still haven't begun to relax yet. We're starting to get a partial idea of what is happening now and what to do next, but I myself have no ideas for an overall plan yet. For now, I at least want to help ease some of the townspeople's anxiety. We were evacuated without knowing anything about what is going on. We were moved. People are starting to argue that we don't even know if we should be here, so we have a lot to talk about from now on. There are man-made aspects to this situation, but if those aspects continue to be taken advantage of as they have been in the mass media, reconstruction will consequently become impossible. What we have to realize is that it would be best to avoid saying that the national government or TEPCO are bad. Our children work at TEPCO, and everyone working on cleaning up this accident is a resident of our town. The townspeople don't really feel like placing the blame on TEPCO. There was an accident, and now they are trying to clean it up. It's less a feeling of blame, and more about just asking for them to do *something*."

Essentially, the people of Futaba are not simply victims of a disaster or accident. Members of their family, husbands and sons, are working to recover from the accident. They are working among deadly levels of radioactive contaminants, dressed in protective clothing, and working their hardest to prevent those materials from spreading. However, the accident has also forced people to live the inconvenient lives of evacuees, so they are surely also victims. Stuck as they are between these two positions, their feelings are complicated.

V. Meeting the Shinsai Shien Network Saitama (SSN)

After our meeting with the deputy mayor, we visited a counseling space set up in a broad hallway. The space had three booths separated by tall partitions and with four pipe chairs set up on either side of a long brown table for a meeting, with those seeking counseling on one side and staff on the other (Figure 4).

A cardboard sign was set up, and someone had drawn some illustrations on it and written the words "The SSN coun-

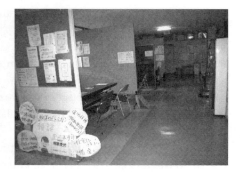

Figure 4. Shinsai Shien Network Saitama counseling space at Kisai High School

seling team is ready to help!" in large characters. It also had a list of likely topics for counseling: employment insurance, labor consultations (unpaid salary), mortgage payments, debt, housing consultations (introduction to properties), living expenses, nuclear accident compensation, bank-related (withdrawals and accounts), reissuing of driver's licenses, and proof of identity. Consultations were being offered every Tuesday, Thursday, and Saturday from 1 to 5 PM.

We waited for the woman at reception to be free before speaking to her. The reception at the counselling booth was being run by a clinical psychologist. Apparently, they were running it under the label "Anything Goes Consultations," and would determine whether or not a person was in need of specialized medical or psychological treatment, then pass them on to the legal specialist in the next booth.

There is a problem with offering such a service titled "Mental health counselling" then having a psychiatrist, psychosomatic specialist, or clinical psychologist sit and wait for someone asking for help in a crowded place with as little privacy as an evacuation center: evacuees find it hard to come. But by offering a service that would "help with any problem you have," a clinical psychologist could receive people in a casual way, working alongside legal and sometimes social welfare specialists. This was a revolutionary idea.

I later heard a story from a group of clinical psychologists from a prefecture in Kanto who had travelled to one of the areas affected by the Tohoku Earthquake to offer "mental health care" support. They had heard that there had been a need for their work so they rushed to the actual place, but they discovered there was nothing they could do. They had heard that Tohoku people are uncomplaining and can endure much, but they said, when they offered their help, people simply responded, "I'm fine. Thank you for doing so much to help us." Apparently many of the groups of clinical psychologists had returned home from the disaster areas after becoming discouraged that they couldn't help. Perhaps this occurred because they arrived at the field wearing a "mental health care staff" nametag and offering to "listen to anything you are worried about." The victims are not mentally ill. They lost everything and they are suffering from their living conditions and economic problems. That is causing a psychological reaction that is resulting in complete exhaustion and anxiety. That is why it is so meaningful to offer "Anything Goes Consultations" support alongside lawyers, judicial scriveners and other legal specialists.

There were six or seven clinical psychologists working to provide volunteer counselling services, and they worked in shifts arranged around their own jobs, three times a week from 1 PM to 5 PM. The service was originally started when there was an evacuation center set up at Saitama Super Arena, and there was a call put out on a mailing list for Saitama school counsellors. Psychologists who could volunteer communicated by email to coordinate which days they could offer their services. When it was thought necessary to follow up with a client, they would mainly share information by telephone. When continuous follow-up care was deemed necessary, they did everything possible to put the client in touch with a specialized institution.

One of the lawyers, Takuo Okamoto, finished a consultation and approached us. We asked him what sorts of questions people were asking at the counselling/consultation booths.

"People have various legal problems, but because they can't actually return home, many people come to us to talk about mental issues, and about difficulties they have living life as evacuees," Okamoto explained. "We also offer practical information they need to live here. For example, we tell them how to receive employment insurance, how to get a license re-issued, from that sort of thing, to individual consultations on what kind of compensation they are entitled to. People are also concerned about problems their children are facing. They had to move schools, and the cultures of Fukushima and Saitama are different, and there are probably differences in the level of scholastic ability as well, so many mothers are worried about whether or not their children will do well here. Most families who brought children have begun moving out of the evacuation center and into each apartment houses, so they have a problem with getting information from the municipalities. For education-related problems, I think it would be good if there was a way for information to be passed between the government and each family through the schools, so right now, I'm struggling to come up with a way of doing that."

The Shinsai Shien Network Saitama (Disaster Support Network Saitama, or SSN) is an organization that was founded on 17 March 2011 after a call from the Anti-Poverty Network Saitama. Around 30 individuals gathered for an emergency meeting, including citizens working in the community to help solve issues related to poverty and suicide, lawyers, and specialists in other fields, and the participants resolved to launch a support network to provide relief to those suffering from the effects of earthquake. Its parent organization, Anti-Poverty Network Saitama, was launched after "The tent city for jobless" had been set up at the end of 2008 in Hibiya Park for temporary workers, to serve as a support network for those living in poverty for a variety of reasons, including the homeless, the unemployed, and those suffering from illness. Members come from all walks of life, and include lawyers, judicial scriveners, and other legal specialists, social workers, clinical psychologists, school teachers, students, and other citizens. It has held consultation sessions both large and small, provided night-time counselling and lectures for citizens, and held gatherings for people concerned to come together and connect.

The Emergency Evacuation Phase   17

On 18 March, they went to the evacuation center at Saitama Super Arena, offered volunteers, and began offering support after coordinating efforts and roles with other organizations. The "Volunteer Station HQ" at Saitama Super Arena was run by the Saitama Prefectural Social Welfare Council. Systematically laid out below them were teams in charge of social workers, volunteer matching, cooking, information, public relations, supplies, and consultation support. The consultation support team was run by the SSN. Information Environment Communications, a general incorporated association run by Yutaka Aiko (which would later join the SSN and become its administrative core), was in charge of the information team. After a request was made to Nippon Telegram and Telephone (NTT) cooperation, a system was built at the evacuation center to offer internet access, and the evacuees could freely make use of the internet when they wished. The staff also hung a sign reading, "We will look up anything you need," and did searches and that sort of thing for the elderly and others unable to find information on their own. They helped evacuees obtain the latest information available, including helping them confirm their immediate family and other relatives were safe, search for relatives at other evacuation centers, find directions to work and secondary evacuation centers, information on the local community, information on children's schools, local government announcements, conditions of local lifeline recovery, procedures for obtaining disaster victim certificates, information on emergency loans, and more. In addition, they said that they also provided support to the public employees of the town of Futaba who had moved to the arena, and helped relaunch the town's website, etc.

The evacuation center at Saitama Super Arena was open for two weeks, from the 17th to the 31st of March, and it housed a maximum of approximately 2,500 evacuees. It is rare to have an urban evacuation center of such an extreme size. The majority of evacuation centers have been located in school gymnasiums and municipal buildings, and it is rare for such a large-scale event facility to be put to such use. With that, it was necessary to implement methods of support that could handle an unprecedented number of people, and every night, the heads of the various volunteer teams would gather for an information exchange meeting. They talked about problems that had occurred and how to deal with them, and how to ensure all could have access to support.

Mr. Okamoto began talking about their comprehensive support plan for the future.

"Of everyone that came together for the arena, right now we have the board of the bar association, judicial scrivener association and clinical psychologist association, and we're talking about how to create a support system for the future. We have already started to move in creating a system that can provide more comprehensive support, talking to the government first, and to professional associations and other private organizations."

18   Part I - 1

After that, the SSN's representative and lawyer Tadashi Inomata finished a long phone call and came over.

"Sorry for making you wait," he said. "My name is Inomata. I was just speaking to the Japanese Red Cross Society (JRCS), who are gathering donations to provide six-item sets of fridges and other appliances for people moving into temporary housing. Right now, the donations are apparently restricted to people moving into temporary housing in Miyagi and Iwate. But the JRCS just told me that if there is similar demand in Saitama, they will be able to help."

The JRCS six-item appliance set includes a washer, refrigerator, television, rice cooker, microwave, and electric kettle. These items are essential not only for those whose homes were destroyed by the earthquake or tsunami to rebuild their lives, but also for those forced to flee their homes due to radioactive contamination. Mr. Inomata says that by properly surveying people's needs and numerically determining where demand lies, it is possible that the social support situation will change.

"I think it is necessary to survey people's needs to adjust the system wherever it is inadequate and to start projects that can provide support. It would be great if we could collaborate on that sort of survey."

It was a welcome offer, and if we could get the cooperation of Futaba, we could do something so meaningful. By clarifying where the evacuee residents were experiencing difficulties in their lives, and learning about the desires of each resident, it might be possible for us to help make their current lives a little better.

"Actually, when we were at Saitama Super Arena, we did a needs survey of a pretty large number of people," Mr. Inomata continued. "We also provided individual consultations, with more than 500 just on life counselling alone. Would you be able to analyze the results we got?"

"So, you have survey data taken from a large sample of people just sitting around, and there is nobody to analyze it? We couldn't ask for more. Thank you very much. We will try out best," I answered.

We were asked to take up two projects: analyze questionnaire data gathered previously, and create a survey to determine people's needs, potentially in collaboration with the SSN and Futaba town in the future. We'd finally found a way to do something for the people affected by the disaster.

VI. Survey plan to solve the problems at the evacuation center

■ 17 May (Tuesday)
I got a phone call from lawyer Tadashi Inomata, the head of SSN. Last week, on Friday the 13th of May, he had received permission to take part in the meeting between the town of Futaba and city of Kazo held weekly at Kisai High School. Mr. Inomata called to ask if we could make up a sample of the questionnaire we had been working on by the meeting next week.

We could sense that Mr. Inomata impatiently wanted us to respond to the request as quickly as possible. In the constantly changing conditions of the evacuation center at Kisai High School, he wanted to improve the living environment in the evacuation center quickly. The issues he was most conscious of were the need for partitions and making it so people could cook for themselves.

Many evacuation centers in East Japan were in the process of having cardboard or curtain partitions installed. It was said that the Cabinet Office's Disaster Volunteer Liaison Desk was also promoting the installation of partitions. As people's stays in the evacuation centers were prolonged, Mr. Inomata believed that the fact that women had no place to change their clothing would be abnormally stressful for them. The other issue was food. Although more than two months had passed since the disaster, the evacuees at Kisai High School were still relying on distributed bento boxes and bread. Mr. Inomata said that the Co-op provided them with freshly made miso soup only once a week, elderly residents were complaining that they couldn't eat only fried food, and many bento boxes were being thrown out. At one point, Futaba Town Office had worked to make it so people could cook for themselves in the school, but sanitary issues led Kazo City's health center to shut that effort down. This situation would lead to enormous problems if it were to continue for more than a year.

Mr. Inomata thought an anonymous questionnaire might allow people to write down the things they couldn't say. If the results showed that a large number of people wanted partitions and the ability to cook, he thought that Kazo City Hall would be forced to respond.

We sped up the work schedule, thought about what the questionnaire should entail, and decided to quickly summarize the whole picture. We consulted with Professor Hiroaki Kumano, a specialist in Clinical Psychology Assessment Studies, and decided to use the Stress Response Scale SRS-18. To determine physical condition, we would use the medical interview questionnaire I had used after the Kobe Earthquake.

Another important thing to assess is living environment. We consulted with Professor Takaya Kojima, a specialist in Architectural Environmental Engineering and decided to use an excerpt from a survey on facility satisfaction compiled by the Ministry of Land, Infrastructure and Transport (MLIT) to measure "work environment comfort." In addition to the above, we wanted to make up a more comprehensive question sheet that would cover food, child-rearing and other lifestyle issues, employment and other economic issues, and disaster compensation and other legal issues.

First of all, however, what was most important was to clearly lay out the objectives of the questionnaire.

Questionnaire Objective
Assess the mental and physical state of residents and problems in living conditions and living environment at present in order to devise policies that will lead to greater safety and comfortability as residents' stays in evacuation centers become more long-term in the future.

The mayor was putting a great effort alongside the staffs of Futaba Town Office to work for the residents of Futaba every day. We did not want to pressure the town office to improve residents' lives based on a questionnaire conducted by an external organization. To the greatest extent possible, we wanted to make Futaba Town Office the main player in conducting the questionnaire to help make the residents' lives better. It was likely that the town itself would want a broader gathering of ideas from the residents. I wanted to incorporate questions on a broad range of subjects so the town office could gather the information it wanted to know about the people of Futaba, and work with the people of the town office to create the survey items.

Next in order of importance, we needed to prepare the environment so that the residents would fully understand the significance of cooperation in our questionnaire survey. For example, we could ask for the cooperation of the leaders of each room and of volunteer staff who had become closely involved with each resident. For elderly residents unable to write on their own, we must think up a way of conducting interviews and writing their responses for them.

We created an overall explanation of the questionnaire to be used in the survey, setting "state of mind and body" as the response variable, and "living situation/environment" and "disaster degree and future forecast" as explanatory variables. We provided that document to Mr. Inomata to present to the meeting between Futaba and Kazo as our proposal for the survey. The proposal was as follows.

The Emergency Evacuation Phase   21

Questionnaire Aim

This questionnaire survey to be carried out mainly by Futaba Town Office is meant to improve living conditions for town residents. It will collect a broad range of information the town office is looking for. Then the town office will actively deal with issues the town office can address, and the results of the survey can be used as a bargaining chip in negotiations with Saitama Prefecture, Fukushima Prefecture, and related ministries for requests regarding other issues.

Assessment Items

(1) Recent physical condition: Medical interview questionnaire used after the Kobe Earthquake
(2) Recent mental condition: Stress Response Scale
(3) Living environment: Excerpt from MLIT facility satisfaction survey
(4) Living conditions: Food questions, childrearing and other lifestyle questions, employment and other economic questions, legal questions, etc.
(5) Disaster degree: distance from the nuclear plant, level of destruction of the building, loss of family, etc.
(6) Future forecast: When does the individual expect that a return to Futaba will be possible? How long will the individual find it possible to live at Kisai High School? Where is the individual considering moving? (Within Fukushima? Within Saitama?)

■ 27 May (Friday)

Fortunately, during the Futaba-Kazo meeting that Mr. Inomata attended, it was decided that the questionnaire survey would be implemented. At the request of the Deputy Mayor, I would participate in the meeting to provide a more detailed explanation of the concrete plan for the survey questionnaire.

The meeting is known as the Kisai High School Volunteer Staff Meeting, and with the permission of Futaba Town Office, people volunteering at Kisai High School's evacuation center held the meeting once a week to share information and to respond to any issues that arise. It was held in the Japanese-style room on the second floor of the Student Hall, and lasted two and a half hours, taking place for two and a half hours, between 16:30 and 19:00. For the meeting, Deputy Mayor Inoue was joined by two volunteer heads from the town office, one person from Futaba Municipal Social Welfare Council, Mr. Yamamoto (pseudonym), the head of Kazo's Health Care Department, three people from the social worker team, and three people from the SSN, including lawyer Tadashi Inomata representing the SSN, a judicial scrivener and the SSN's deputy representative named Hirose, and myself, for a total of ten people.

Mr. Yamamoto stated that without seeing the issues directly, support could not be provided, and said that he had visited the evacuation center at Kisai High School every day for the first 40 days it had been open. An acupuncture volunteer stated that the number of residents receiving massages was dropping and was expected to continue dropping into June. In other words, from his point of view, the acute period had passed, residents' lives had more or less settled down, and the need for volunteers had decreased. In contrast, lawyer Tadashi Inomata from the SSN reported that resident anxiety and stress levels were at their limit.

"We at the SSN are providing 'Anything Goes Consultations' through the volunteer efforts of clinical psychologists, lawyers, and judicial scriveners," Mr. Inomata told those gathered for the meeting. "Recently, the time of each consultation has been increasing. Conversations never end, people's anxiety and stress are rising, and there are people ready to explode from the stress of relationship and employment problems, and people who have completely shut down. As fast as we can, we need to improve the environment they are living in."

At this stage, Mr. Inomata asserted, in order to determine what needs to be done to improve the environment, a survey of the residents' needs was required. They had been living in the evacuation center for almost two months. Had the conditions stabilized or had they gotten worse? At the very least, it was clear that the evacuation center was moving into the next phase. It was necessary to gain an objective understanding of how the situation was progressing.

Later, the discussion turned to the questionnaire survey. First, I used a draft of the questionnaire to explain the survey's objectives, methods, and specific items that the survey would cover. One of the social workers helping with elderly and infant care at the evacuation center voiced doubts about the accuracy, saying, "Is it possible to understand the infinite variety of problems people face in a questionnaire targeting a large group of people?" This individual seems to have had the impression that the survey could cause agitation at the high school.

It is true that a questionnaire is more directed at uncovering group problems than individual problems, so I answered, "By adding a place for people to write freely, we think we can get a slightly better idea of more individual issues. However, by getting a more comprehensive picture of the situation through numerical values, we think the town will get a better idea of what measures to take."

It was important for the questionnaire to address that impression of potential disturbance at the evacuation center. It was essential to communicate why the survey was being conducted and for whom, to avoid the survey simply becoming a "survey for the sake of a survey," conducted by those in power. As much as possible, we had to come up with items that would help the residents, and then once the survey was complete, communicate the results to them and devise and implement measures that reflected those results.

Mayor Idogawa's intention was to implement the questionnaire with all residents of Futaba. It would be conducted from late June into July. One individual suggested that four types of questionnaire could be made up. They would have shared items and items particular to understanding the characteristics of the regions in which the evacuation centers were located. There were four main areas which the approximately 7,000 residents of Futaba had evacuated. There were around 1,000 living together at the Kisai High School evacuation center, and 700 living together at the Listel Inawashiro evacuation center in the Aizu area of Fukushima Prefecture. Third were the approximately 1,800 people living individually in locations throughout Fukushima, and fourth were the approximately 3,500 people living in other prefectures outside of Fukushima. The questionnaire would be administered by the town, the results would be managed by the town, and in principle, the town's intention was that the results could not be used for any other purpose. This survey was not to be conducted for academic reasons, and the results were not to be released in a paper. Our task was to develop a survey questionnaire that would be, to the greatest extent possible, answer the needs of the people living in the evacuation centers.

As the meeting that day came to an end, all the participants shared their opinions, and the idea for a cooperative framework was floated, through which question items that helped the residents could be created. Using the questionnaire we had made as a foundation, it was decided that the subject would undergo further review the following week, and the meeting was closed.

■ 10 June (Friday)
Based on the cooperation of Futaba Town Office, the content of the questionnaire survey of the residents created by the SSN and Waseda University had at last been finalized. Then in June, I received a phone call from Deputy Mayor Inoue.

"I'm sorry. Due to various circumstances, it has been decided that implementation of the questionnaire survey must be delayed. We recognize all the hard work you put into it, and must sincerely apologize."

He said that Mayor Idogawa had made the decision for various reasons. What could it have been? We later discovered that there was an incident in which a man living at Kisai High School was arrested for having engaged in deplorable actions at the evacuation center. The mayor felt deeply responsible that one of the residents of the town could be arrested in that way. With trust in the town having been lost, it is possible that they thought the timing for carrying out the scheduled questionnaire survey might be poor.

Whatever the case may be, the questionnaire that we had spent a sleepless month or so preparing suddenly went in vain. Both the SSN's Inomata and I were, naturally, deeply disappointed. However, there was nothing that could be done. This was the result of the emergency situation caused by the earthquake and nuclear power plant disaster. When the questionnaire is undertaken by the town of Futaba, it has to be conducted at a time good for the town office, or it will have no meaning, and following that, will serve for no purpose for the residents of Futaba either. The purpose of the survey is to find ways to improve the living environment of people who have been evacuated due to the nuclear power plant accident, and to the last, we support the town of Futaba.

VII. Implementing the survey

It was in this way that the cancelled questionnaire survey would be implemented in a different form one year after the disaster in March of 2012.

At the suggestion of the Disaster Relief Office at the Saitama Bar Association, including lawyer Takuo Okamoto, who I had met at Kisai High School, the Saitama Disaster Measures Liaison Council was formed in May 2011, to coordinate victim support activities undertaken by government bodies and private organizations in Saitama Prefecture. Saitama Prefecture's Crisis and Disaster Management Department, Saitama Social Welfare Department Policy Division and the like joined the council, as did more than ten municipal governments from the prefecture; seven professional organizations, including the social worker association, clinical psychologist association, judicial scrivener association, and tax accountant association; and 12 private support organizations, including the SSN and Information Environment Communications. Almost 50 members in total came together and began holding monthly committee meetings (Figure 5).

The sixth meeting took place on the 20th of December, and it was decided that the liaison council would itself undertake to plan and conduct a questionnaire survey of the 5,000 evacuees living in Saitama to recognize the year that had passed since the disaster and determine what measures could be taken in the future. The SSN, and we at Waseda University, were put in charge of survey administration, and we began creating the questionnaire form. In order to create the questionnaire, we gathered opinions and ideas from all of the council's member organizations about current issues and problems and about information they needed to clarify in order to imple-

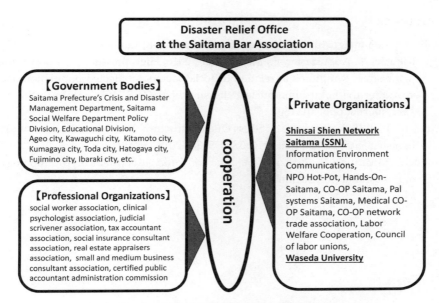

Figure 5. Members of Saitama Disaster Measures Liaison Council

ment support programs. Moreover, we also held multiple meetings on creating question items with lawyers, judicial scriveners, clinical psychologists, and social workers providing support on site, and with several people affected by the disaster. At Waseda University, a collaborative research team was formed between my Medical Anthropology laboratory, Professor Hiroaki Kumano's Clinical Psychology Assessment laboratory, and Assistant Professor Kazutaka Masuda's Gerontological Social Welfare laboratory.

The objectives of the questionnaire survey were to (1) gain an understanding of current conditions for victims, (2) examine how to provide future support, and (3) to make recommendations to the government. The survey was implemented at 1,658 evacuating households throughout Saitama Prefecture in March 2012. The results of the survey have been shared with the Disaster Measures Liaison Council, published in newspapers, reported in the TV news, presented in the NHK special and other television programs, and have been used in written arguments presented to the Nuclear Damage Compensation Dispute Reconciliation Center and in court cases connected to judgements on the nuclear power plant accident. More details on the results can be found in the English-language journal PLOS ONE (2016), and in my contribution to the second part of this publication.

Reference

Tsujiuchi, T., Yamaguchi, M., Masuda, K., Tsuchida, M., Inomata, T., Kumano, H., Kikuchi, Y., Augusterfer, E., Mollica, R.F., 2016. High prevalence of post-traumatic stress symptoms in relation to social factors in affected population one year after the Fukushima nuclear disaster. *PLoS ONE* 11(3), e0151807. doi:10.1371/journal.pone.0151807.

Tsujiuchi, T., 2019. Post-traumatic Stress Due to Structural Violence after Fukushima Disaster. *Japan Forum*, doi:10.1080/09555803.2018.1552308.

Tsujiuchi, T., Masuda, K., 2019. *Fukushima no iryō jinrui gaku.* [Medical Anthropology of Fukushima.], Tōmi Shobō.

---

* This paper is a record of the fieldwork I conducted in the approximately three months after the Fukushima Nuclear Power Plant accident in March 2011. It is an ethnographic report on how we as university research institution could support the victims of the disaster, and the steps we took to intervene in the disaster area. It depicts how we came up with a survey research method that could be of use to the field through the cooperation of victims, supporters, and other researchers.

2 Mental Health / Community Health / Social well-being

How to Practice Social Care by Collaboration between several professionality

Multi-vocal Analysis of Supporters

Jihye Kim CP, MA[1][4] *(Clinical Psychology),*
Kazutaka Masuda CSW, PhD[2][4] *(Studies of Social Work),*
Takuya Tsujiuchi MD, PhD[3][4] *(Medical Anthropology),*
Shinsai Shien Network Saitama (SSN)

Key words: inter-professional collaboration, social care, social support,
Fukushima nuclear accident, multi-vocal analysis

I. Introduction

This paper aims to paint a clearer, multifaceted view of multidisciplinary social care proffered through collaboration with experts in psychology, social welfare, law, and a diverse range of other specialized fields. To do so, we present the opinions of six members of the Shinsai Shien Network Saitama (SSN), an organization that has been offering disaster relief since the 2011 Tohoku earthquake. The authors are a part of a team from Waseda University involved in the operation of the SSN, with specific contributions including the analysis of survey data on victim needs, development of questionnaires aimed at evacuees, and other survey and research efforts.

The parent organization of the SSN is the Saitama Anti-Poverty Network (APN). The APN was formed after the issue of contract worker layoffs called "Haken-giri" in Japanese came to light at the end of 2008 with the incident that resulted in the founding of the New Year Dispatch Village. The network formed for the purpose of resolv-

---

*1 Division of Clinical Psychology, Graduate School of Education, The University of Tokyo
*2 Lecturer, Department of Psychology and Social Welfare, School of Letters, Mukogawa Women's University
*3 Professor, Faculty of Human Sciences, Waseda University
*4 Waseda Institute of Medical Anthropology on Disaster Reconstruction (WIMA)

ing poverty issues on both the societal and political levels, to help secure basic human living needs and guarantee employment. The staff of the APN is truly diverse, made up of lawyers, judicial scriveners, clinical psychologists, and social workers – including former recipients of social welfare – and includes citizens, students, and labor unions working on poverty issues. The APN offers help with economic poverty, but also provides counselling for low-income individuals suffering from "relationship poverty" due to their isolation from the rest of society. It holds consultation sessions both large and small, night patrol counseling, civic lectures, and gatherings to bring individuals in similar situations together to have the chance to connect.

After the nuclear accident in March 2011 caused by the Tohoku earthquake, thousands of people, primarily from Fukushima Prefecture, fled to Saitama Prefecture. APN leader Tadashi Inomata called an emergency meeting of around 30 individuals, including lawyers, various specialists, and citizens who worked in the community on a daily basis to resolve poverty issues, help prevent people from passing away alone, and more. It was there that the Shinsai Shien Network was launched to provide evacuees with disaster relief, and relief operations began at the enormous evacuation center set up in Saitama Super Arena, where more than 2,500 people had fled. For information on the situation on the ground at that time, and on how the team at Waseda University became involved with the SSN, please see Part I, Chapter 1, titled, "The Emergency Evacuation Phase: Fieldwork on nuclear accident evacuee support in Saitama."

The six individuals introduced in this chapter include a lawyer, a judicial scrivener, a clinical psychologist, a system engineer, a social worker, and a specialist in labor welfare. They met at Saitama Super Arena and, through providing disaster relief, built a collaborative framework that harnessed the expertise of each individual. I believe that the synergistic effect of these fields of expertise coming together squared their effectiveness, essentially creating a network that was 6 X 6 36 time more effective than it would have been had they all been working as individuals. How do those individuals look back on the disaster relief efforts aimed at the nuclear plant victims? In this chapter, we will look carefully at the concept of multidisciplinary social care from the perspective of these six individuals.

II. Interview procedure

The interviews were conducted three years after the earthquake and subsequent nuclear accident in the summer and autumn of 2014. In preparation for the interviews, we asked the informants to let the student interviewers visit the locations where they were volunteering and take part in their relief work. This was meant to give the interviewers a better understanding of what sort of relief the interviewees provided and the atmosphere in which they worked, and it would help them build a relationship with the interviewees. Our research project leader, Tsujiuchi, was also on the SSN steering committee, and had already built relationships with these individuals after collaborating with them in providing relief operations over the three years since the disaster.

We then drew up an interview request letter describing in concrete terms the objective and method of the interviews, describing how their privacy would be protected, and detailing how the results of the information gathered during the interviews would be used. At that time, a list of the main questions the interviewers wanted to ask each interviewee was formulated based on the experiences the interviewers gained while engaged in the relief work, and this was appended to the interview request letter.

The actual interviews were conducted by the students in one-on-one direct meetings with the interviewees. One of our major goals was, to the greatest extent possible, get the real opinions of the individuals providing disaster relief, which is why we thought it important for the interviewers to carefully listen to the narratives offered freely during the discussions, so there was an attempt made to ensure the interviews were conducted in a free-talk format. The conversations were recorded on a digital voice recorder with the consent of the interviewees.

After the interviews, the audio data was transcribed into text format verbatim. Verbal information was included when creating the transcriptions, but non-verbal information provided by the interviewees was also included in text form, based on interviewer notes taken during the interviews and their recollections. This was in an attempt to gain a realistic image of how the actual interview went.

When the transcriptions were completed, the text was edited to make it easier to understand, with explanations added to clarify proper nouns and dialect terms. Moreover, the interviews were separated into sections, and subheadings were added to correspond with the themes that arose. Once the edits, additions, and subheadings were completed, the transcripts were sent to each interviewee to have the content checked, and they were asked to remove any details that may intrude on any individual's personal privacy and to add any explanations they felt were needed.

We rewrote the transcription data obtained through the above process in prose to make it easier for the reader to understand. At the same time, we extracted statements that were important to portraying the experience of the interviewees, and other sections were replaced with explanatory text. When this rewrite process was complete, the content was again sent to all interviewees, who provided a final check to ensure there were no factual errors or privacy issues.

III. Informant Profiles

1. Tadashi Inomata (Lawyer)

Inomata described the perspective that led him to decide to become a lawyer. "People find happiness in their relationships with other people...but it's not about waiting passively for relationships to be made – happiness comes from actively grasping the moment yourself" he said. "Through your actions, you can get involved with helping people in trouble get back on their feet. I am always thankful whenever I get to see someone's eyes light up for the first time in a long while."

As a lawyer, Inomata has worked on multi-debt relief issues and other problems related to consumer damages, but as the multiple debt problem became a more serious social issue, he turned his efforts to the poverty that lay at the root of those debt problems. Before the earthquake, Inomata joined the Poverty Reduction Office at the Japan Federation of Bar Associations and the Metropolitan Welfare Support Lawyers' Network, where he worked to improve the system dealing with issues such as irregular contract work and welfare and provide support activities where they were needed. Dispatch worker layoffs became a society-wide problem at the end of 2008, when the New Year Dispatch Workers Village was opened in Hibiya and around 500 dispatch workers and other people travelled from around the country to stay there in Hibiya Park. Inomata took charge of life counselling services in the dispatch village, stayed there day after day, and helped many dispatch workers. In addition, since 2009, he followed through with the former citizens of the dispatch worker village who had dealt with psychological, employment, and life issues. As a member of the APN, he also continued to provide the same counselling and support services he'd offered at the dispatch village within Saitama Prefecture. The earthquake evacuees faced the same situation as the laid-off dispatch workers in that they had lost both their jobs and their homes at the same instant. The efforts at the dispatch village and the APN led to the formation of the SSN, and from there to the subsequent counselling and support services.

Inomata is a lawyer with a gentle demeanor, but he refuses to forgive the various injustices of modern society, and he carries within him a burning passion for social change. He listens carefully to others and thoroughly avoids pushing his own ideas. In that way, he is able to bring around even the most argumentative people and encourage them to be a bit more flexible without them even noticing. In addition, Inomata has a sharp nose for sniffing out what someone needs "right now", even within constantly changing situations. The authors have continued to work with Inomata, fully trusting that we can make no mistakes if we follow the path he has laid.

How to Practice Social Care by Collaboration between several professionality   31

The provision of disaster relief on site is fraught with various difficulties and continuously appearing barriers, and there were numerous times arguments both within the team and with people outside of the team. However, Inomata's tenacity and ability to maintain a dialogue ensured that the SSN has remained on course and continues to provide support today.

2. Takashi Hirose (Judicial Scrivener)

Hirose graduated from the Faculty of Law at Waseda University and took up a regular office job. He says, in the past, he had had an interest in working with the needy, but after joining a company, he was no longer free to do such support work. He didn't want to work for himself – he wanted to spend his life working for other people and for society, so he decided to become a judicial scrivener.

As a judicial scrivener, Hirose worked often with individuals having difficulties maintaining the basic needs of life and began thinking about how best to offer such individuals support. That is when he realized that, "It's not enough to solve the problems we see bubbling up and then end our support." Also, Hirose describes what he calls "real support" as not simply solving the problems individuals are directly facing. Real support must also take into consideration the emotional state of the needy and provide social resources and security after the problems have been resolved. Therefore, he regularly works with recipients of social welfare, with monthly night patrols conducted to uncover the opinions of people living on the streets and encourage them to receive welfare, and holding gatherings in order to help protect against isolation for people looking for employment after going on social welfare support. Hirose is skilled at lightening the atmosphere with gentle jokes, is always humble, and can pinpoint people's strong points. He is capable of providing support under any circumstances. Disaster victims are also able to speak with Hirose about their legal woes and worries about maintaining a livelihood, and when they do, they seem to find themselves feeling a bit better and their hopes rekindled.

3. Yuko Hagiwara (Clinical Psychologist)

"I had a difficult experience when I was young," Hagiwara told us. "And I was able to overcome it through the help of people who listened to my troubles and gave me support." Here gratitude for that help changed the way she thought. "I wanted to do something to help people who were facing difficult times alone," she said. That led her to obtain her certification as a clinical psychologist, and she began providing mental support to elderly individuals, primarily through psychological education and examinations, and through reminiscence therapy. After the earthquake, a senior colleague told Hagiwara about the volunteer work being done by the Saitama Society of Certified Clinical Psychologists, and Hagiwara joined the SSN's efforts. Hagiwara says that she continues to work as a volunteer to "be there for people, help them get what they need, and do my utmost to give them what they are looking for." At social gatherings and consultation sessions for disaster victims, Hagiwara has the wondrous ability to give people a sense of safety and security without ever having to emphasize her expertise as a clinical psychologist. At evacuation centers, she gave victims hand massages, handed out tea and snacks at get-togethers, and generally helped people with their mental health in a natural, unobtrusive way. We believe that this attitude is the ideal attitude for a clinical psychologist working in disaster relief.

4. Yu Aiko (Systems Engineer)

Yu Aiko heads the SSN offices and is the representative of an IT company called Information Environment Communications. The company was founded on philosophy of providing problem resolution through communications in an improved information environment, and the company primarily works to support lawyers and judicial scriveners through more efficient business operations and information sharing made possible through cloud computing and other means. Aiko was also laid off, when the company he had worked at for many years since graduating university was bought up after the bankruptcy of the Lehman Brothers sent shockwaves through the world's economy. He knew that he had to do something for himself, and just when he began to think about starting his own company – one that wouldn't be about competition but about contributing to the community as much as was possible –, the earthquake struck Tohoku and the nuclear power plant accident occurred. The timing was perfect for Aiko. "There were people in need around me," he said. "And I knew I had to do my best to help, whatever it was." That thought process led him to get involved in disaster relief. Every year, Aiko harnesses the many skills he has honed over the years – planning, activity, writing, presentations, and negotiations – when he visits various organizations to obtain subsidies, and he is an absolutely indispensable part of SSN operations. As the head of the offices, he has taken the lead in practical planning and management at the SSN.

5. Akihiro Takano (Social Worker)

Takano is a social worker who has lived a stormy life, having lived on the streets and having received welfare. He decided to retire at 45 from the major department store he'd worked at for 26 years in order to care for his father, who had been diagnosed with cancer. He had difficulty finding work after his father passed away, and from August 2009, he was forced to live on the streets at the age of 54. After living homeless for three and a half months, he started to receive welfare, but describes the time as having been "very difficult, with many recruiters refusing to help me due to my age." However, for him, "it was a chance for me to start again with a new life." After that difficult period, Takano took on his current position, where he harnesses his own experiences as a member of the Anti-Poverty Network in Saitama. When a request for help comes in from a needy individual, Takano arranges food and immediately rushes to the location. He listens to the stories of the needy, recommends they apply for social welfare, introduces them to legal offices and NPOs that provide consultations on public assistance, and even accompanies such individuals to public offices to help them apply. He has also worked with the SSN since the Tohoku earthquake. Takano has one foot firmly planted in the practical aspects of his job. He has experienced the difficulties that life can throw at us and survived, which is why he is able to do the delicate social work he does.

6. Nobuo Nagata (Labor and Welfare Council)

Nagata is Senior Managing Director at the Saitama Labor and Welfare Council. The principle underlying the practice of labor welfare comes from the post-war era, when Japan suffered from severe supply shortages, and the goal was, as a nation, to procure daily necessities for workers and provide more stability in their lives. With that background, Nagata has worked in various activities designed to stabilize the lives of people working in the local community, from giving consultations on labor, debt, law, taxes, pension, life planning, housing and other issues, to providing support in finding employment, child-rearing, and nursing care, and offering motivational support. In addition, through his work, he has built relationships with experts, local governments, management groups, cooperatives, and various types of NPO, and has strong ties to government and professional organizations. He made effective use of those ties while providing disaster relief in response to the 2011 Tohoku earthquake. Nagata's broad network and inherent magnanimity allowed him to promptly gather necessary relief supplies from different areas for victims in the constantly changing conditions after the disaster struck. He is skilled at coordinating people in groups both large and small to maintain the harmony, and he has earned the trust of the leaders of mutual aid victim groups providing support around Saitama Prefecture.

IV. Support efforts at Saitama Super Arena

On March 18, 2011, one week after the earthquake, around 1,600 people evacuated from the coastal areas of Fukushima Prefecture to Saitama Super Arena. Even though much time has passed, the memories of that tragic time have remained fresh in the minds of the supporters we interviewed for this paper, and they described the situation for us.

"The evacuees at the Super Arena had to sleep in the hallways on cardboard and other items. and at first, there was no way to partition off space, so they had no privacy," Inomata said. "Many of the evacuees didn't have the time to grab any money or a change of clothes, and had fled with just the clothes on their backs. We had people who were separated from their families, people who were sick or injured, and people who had run away in fear after hearing the explosions at the nuclear power plant."

"There was nothing at the arena at all; they had just offered the space itself," Hirose said. "We couldn't go in the main hall because part of the ceiling had collapsed, so everyone was crowded together to sleep in the hallways, where there was no space to even walk. People of all ages lived there for almost two weeks, from babies to grandmothers in their late-80s."

"It was a nightmare," explained Hagiwara. "I couldn't imagine how such a thing could actually happen. After the nuclear accident, people had moved from evacuation center to evacuation center before finally being brought to Saitama. They thought they would be able to return home , and so they remained restless and unsettled all crammed together in those narrow spaces. It's hard to express in words, but it was like a whirlpool of negativity, with emotions running from confusion to anger."

In these tragic circumstances, these individuals developed the support they provided by considering what to prioritize when, and thinking about what they themselves could offer.

1. Implementation of Needs Survey

As a lawyer and SSN representative, Inomata knew that it was necessary to understand the difficulties and conditions being directly faced by the evacuees living in the large-scale shelter before they could offer consultations and other support services. In order to accomplish that, groups of two to three SSN members conducted a survey of evacuee needs by moving around the arena asking the evacuees about the difficulties they were having, their health, what supplies they needed, etc. The results of that survey were used to provide a broad range of support that harnessed their diverse expertise.

Some of the results of the survey were sent over to the Cabinet Office in response to a request for cooperation. The research team at Waseda University has worked with the SSN since its formation, and in the last seven years, we have conducted annual large-scale questionnaire surveys targeting thousands and even tens of thousands of individuals (Tsujiuchi, T., et al., 2016). The questionnaires covered items such as living conditions, economic situation, employment status, residential environment, physical condition, lifestyle habits, mental condition and stress levels, and how subjects are responding to radiation exposure. This information has clarified the changing needs of people in the years that have passed since the disaster struck, and has been very useful in providing support services. The results of these surveys are discussed in Part II in Tsujiuchi's paper in Chapter 2, Iwagaki's paper in Chapter 3,

Masuda's paper in Chapter 4, Taga's paper in Chapter 5, and Ishikawa's paper in Chapter 8.

Aiko told us about the importance of conducting the large-scale survey.

"Everyone is different, and the problems they face are different too, so it's really important to have numerical data that gives us an overall understanding of the situation," Aiko explained. "The results were pretty close to how we felt on site. In a way, the survey was meant to test our hypothesis, and we were able to verify that hypothesis with the data we received. Some things need data, for example post-traumatic stress disorder (PTSD). We got an objective and quantitative understanding of people's emotional trauma using psychological tests. In order to get the government and the political machinery moving, we had to have that kind of convincing, objective data. I believe that is really important."

2. Establishing the Open Consultation desk

Inomata believed that it was necessary to meet the needs uncovered by the survey and continue conducting it, and he called in the help of various specialists, from lawyers and other legal experts, to clinical psychologists, social workers, mental health care workers, educational experts, and labor unions. This allowed them to begin offering consultation services to respond to various issues.

The consultation desk was staffed by a clinical psychologist, who listened to the various worries and troubles being carried by the evacuees who visited the desk. The clinical psychologists assessed their issues as they spoke and would then guide those seeking help to the appropriate expert. Because there was a variety of expertise on offer, the helpers were split into teams, with the lawyers and judicial scriveners handling issues relating to life and the law, the social workers taking over when nursing care or a welfare response was needed, and the clinical psychologists handling the response when mental health care was deemed necessary.

Hagiwara is our team's clinical psychologist, and she was in charge of receiving people at the Open Consultation desk. She naturally provided mental health care, but she also told us that many people were struggling with more immediate living problems like finding a home and money. Therefore, it was necessary for her to serve as a bridge between the evacuees and the experts, and help the evacuees find the help that best suited their needs.

"Most people find it hard to spell out the issues they are facing in simple words, so with a clinical psychologist on the front desk, they could take their time telling us their story, and I would do my best to help them organize their thoughts and see what they wanted to know. I would then connect them to the judicial scrivener or lawyer they needed," Hagiwara explained.

The consultation desk had more than 100 people a day coming when we were at our busiest. People visited for consultations about various issues and worries, and around half were mental health problems. However, there were many individuals dealing with more immediate, life-threatening situations, such as how to secure the money they needed to live. As a judicial scrivener, Hirose offered his expertise for consultations on legal matters, and he explained what the situation was like.

"The consultations people were seeking were less about law and more about money," Hirose told us. "People had money in credit unions in Fukushima, but they hadn't brought their bankbook or bank card, and they had no personal ID or seal to get their money out. In other words, they had no money to live. Everyone was desperate."

Hirose felt that it was important to harness what they learned during these operations in the future, so he sent reports and request forms for the survey to Saitama Prefecture.

"We had different information flying all around us, consultants were being switched in and out, and everybody didn't have the same knowledge. So, I made an informational booklet, a manual, and distributed it for everyone to share. It described the consultation process, information on where specific municipal functions for towns in Fukushima had been relocated, which banks people could get money out of, that sort of thing. I think it will be a good reference for the next large-scale disaster, so I'm keeping it safe."

In addition, there were allegedly a number of women sexually assaulted in the evacuation centers, so a women's only desk was set up, and consultants experienced in women's issues provided hand massages and they listened to the evacuees who visited them. The needs survey and consultation services were offered every day from morning until 21:00 in the evening, and meetings were held with the entire staff before and after.

"Everyone got together every day and talked about the needs survey results, reported on comments they'd received from evacuees, and decided what to do next," Inomata said. "We shared information like 'I met someone dealing with this situation today,'or 'I'm having a problem with this,' or 'Someone needs that.' That kind of information showed us what kind of information would be needed and what support should be offered in the future."

"We had meetings every day before we started and after we finished," Hirose said. "During the morning meetings, we talked about the most urgent problems, like the response to medical issues such as people who needed dialysis and people with dietary restrictions, mortgage problems, and issues with children. In the evening meeting, we reviewed the day. The biggest meeting we had was with 90 people."

This Open Consultation desk was operated for 13 days until the end of March, when the evacuation center at Saitama Super Arena was closed. More than 800 experts lent their support in providing consultation services a total of 1349 times.

3. Information-related needs and response

During the needs surveys and support efforts, it became clear that there was a need for various types of information, including special government measures being announced one after another, a means of confirming the safety of family members in the disaster area, the names of people who had evacuated to Saitama, and what sort of support could be obtained. The information team was created to solve that problem, and they used the internet to provided information gathering and communication services designed to meet those needs.

Aiko negotiated with the contractor who installed phone lines in the evacuation center to set up a public telephone, and successfully had the contractor install an internet connection as well. Following that, he obtained 11 computers from an IT support company that had been founded only six months previously and built an internet corner in the evacuation center which allowed the evacuees to access the internet and obtain various types of information. However, many of the elderly evacuees were unfamiliar with using computers, and it was necessary to devise a means of passing on necessary information to such individuals.

"When you are an elderly person, you may have a lot of things that you want to know but you can't search for that information yourself," Aiko said. "So, I made a cardboard sign to hang on my back while I walked around. It read 'We can search for everything on the internet. Let us know if you need help.' We had 186 volunteers there to help us, and they looked up anything the evacuees wanted to know and helped them learn how to use the computers themselves. Before long, Fuji Xerox had heard about what we were doing, and provided us with printers so we could print out the information and hand it to the people to take with them."

There was no reception desk at the evacuation center and the evacuees kept coming, with numbers peaking at around 2,500 individuals. There wasn't sufficient communication about the situations faced by evacuees in the center or about support information, so the SSN made up a questionnaire to find out exactly who was where. We used that to make an evacuee register that included their names and original addresses, and where they were located within the evacuation center.

Takano provided consultation services as a social worker, and to ensure as many evacuees as possible could get information on the situation as it changed daily, he started a newspaper to communicate the shared needs of the evacuees.

"The situation in the consultation booths was changing all the time," Takano explained. "I thought maybe there was something we could do to take a more active role in giving people the information they needed, rather than just waiting for people to come to us. So, I started handing out a hand-written newspaper. Bank information was most commonly included, and I also included information about the open consultation desk and about housing that was available for free."

4. Interactions between evacuees and supporters

As a side project, the information team created a large message board they called the Fuku-Tama Board in an effort to promote interactions between the peoples of Fukushima and Saitama. On it was posted messages of appreciation from Fukushima evacuees to the people of Saitama and messages offering encouragement from residents of Saitama. The many messages posted to the Fuku-Tama Board provided the volunteers with a lot of encouragement and motivation. Inomata had in his records the following message from a woman in her 30s who had evacuated from Iwaki City.

It read, "I had no idea if the people close to me were safe, and my fear about the nuclear plant made life a living hell. I was so scared when the lifelines were cut because I have a young child, and I was mentally exhausted when I learned about the arena, and I was able to find a spot here. I was worried evacuating to Saitama, where I have no relatives, but I received a warm welcome from the people of Saitama. 'Don't worry,' they told me. 'Iwaki will surely get back on its feet again,' they said, and I will never forget the powerful encouragement their words gave me. Watching the volunteers working as hard as they can, I realized that someday I want to do the same thing to help others. It was hard to lose so much in the earthquake, and many sad things have happened. However, the relationships I have made here in Saitama, and the compassion I have been shown, could never be destroyed in an earthquake or tsunami. They are very important to me. I am so grateful to all the people of Saitama Prefecture."

When the six supporters profiled here look back on their work at Saitama Super

Arena, they tell us that they met a lot of people, but their experience goes beyond just that of the relationship between "supporter" and "supported." They learned the importance of helping each other, and the joy that can be obtained through doing so.

V. Support efforts at Kisai High School

When the Saitama Super Arena evacuation center was shut down at the end of March 2011, evacuees there were dispersed among public facilities and other buildings throughout Saitama Prefecture or moved to apartments as families. In principle, the decision on where they would go was left up to each individual, but around 1,400 evacuees from the town of Futaba were moved to Kisai High School in Kazo City, under the leadership of then-mayor, Katsutaka Idogawa. Kisai High School was a prefectural high school that had been closed since 2008.

Hirose described the high school at the time as being as miserable as the situation at the Super Arena, being "completely without privacy or anything else," but conditions gradually changed. As many as 1,500 people had evacuated to the high school, but the number of people finding new living arrangements through subsidized housing and other means slowly began to grow. In addition, the consultations also changed from urgent issues like people being unable to withdraw money, to more long-term issues regarding getting compensation or making use of the guardianship system."

The relief volunteers continued to provide the same services they had at the Super Arena, including consultations, and information gathering and disseminations, but came to realize the necessity of conducting follow-ups with the people who had moved away from the evacuation center.

1. Implementation and changes to the Open Consultation service

When the evacuees moved to evacuation centers around Saitama Prefecture, we provided consultation services at evacuation centers in Kazo, Kawaguchi, Toro, and other areas. At Kisai High School in Kazo, we set up partitions, tables, and chairs in a space in a hallway to create three booths for consultations. A clinical psychologist was in charge of receiving people, and lawyers provided their consultation services in the booths.

Takano focused the efforts of the Kisai High School consultation desk by operating three days a week, on Tuesdays, Thursdays, and Saturdays. The consultation team had six members, two lawyers, two judicial scriveners, and two clinical psychologists, while Takano served as a coordinator, patrolling the high school, approaching people who seemed to be in need of help, and when desired, directing them to the consultation desk. An average of less than 18 consultations were provided each day, with full use being made of the limited time frame available, from 1,300 to 1,700 each day. Takano explained that even for people from the same town, differences in lifestyle and habits led to trivial but repeated disputes under the stress of living as evacuees. At first glance, people's lives seemed to be settling down, but many evacuees had begun feeling backed into a corner both physically and mentally as, on a daily basis, they dealt with the onset of dementia symptoms with the change of living environment, emotional anxiety due to continued separation from families, and other issues.

2. Implementing follow-up services to prevent isolation

As mentioned above, the consultation desk at Kisai High School's evacuation center was operated three times a week at first, but as the number of people moving out of the evacuation center increased, that was dropped to one day a week. While the number of people finding their own residences to live in was increasing, some people were unable to find a place to live and were left behind in the evacuation center, and Hagiwara was somewhat worried about those individuals. In addition, there were times when individuals who had moved away from the center returned for visits and had to leave again without meeting anyone. Inomata began to explore options that would allow them to provide follow-up consultations as the evacuees dispersed in order to prevent people from feeling isolated.

"We could keep an eye on people when they were living communally in the evacuation center and ask them what they needed, which helped us understand the issues they were having," Inomata explained. "Also, when everyone was in one place, it was easier to provide the information and supplies they needed. But once everyone started leaving the center and they became spread out all over, it was harder to see what they needed, and we couldn't provide information or supplies even when we wanted to for various reasons, because we didn't know where they lived, and that sort of thing."

Inomata wanted to find a solution to this added problem of how to provide care for people who needed a social safety net, so he collaborated with the Saitama Bar Association and Saitama Judicial Scrivener's Association and patiently continued to press everyone about the necessity of providing follow-up consultations. This resulted in an agreement being reached with the Futaba Town Office, and the SSN began to participate in the meetings of the "social welfare team" and follow-ups conducted by Futaba's Social Welfare Council and the Deputy-Mayor.

Inomata felt that to prevent people from feeling isolated, they needed to know where people were, so he began actively visiting the smaller evacuation centers away from

Kisai High School and participating in "consultation patrols." The Disaster Relief Liaison Committee was comprised of individuals in municipal governments throughout Saitama Prefecture, professional groups like the Saitama Judicial Scrivener's Association, and private-sector relief groups likes the SSN and Waseda University, and Inomata actively proposed to the committee that a Consultation Café be established. The café would serve as a place for the evacuees around Saitama to visit freely and enjoy a cup of tea as they spoke with others from their home of Fukushima. In addition, when problems arose, people would be able to quickly consult with the available experts.

3. Disaster Help Line

The Disaster Help Line was operated for three days from June 16, 2011, with the goal of providing various everyday life consultations to help prevent isolation among the evacuees living around Saitama. The help line received a large number of calls from people having issues obtaining information from their town office about receiving donations or getting permission for a temporary return to their homes. They had difficulty getting through to the office by phone, and the website offered only limited information. It was a little under three months after the disaster, and the town had no information provision system in place. In addition, the help line received a number of calls from individuals with supply issues, including from one who had found an apartment but was without furniture because the six-piece furniture sets that were meant to be provided by the Japanese Red Cross Society (JRCS) had not arrived.

The scars of the disaster were still raw for some, and many people were living isolated lives in areas they were not familiar with, so Hirose was particularly worried about the dangers of suicide among the evacuees. He told us one story about one evacuee who was isolated and suffering and contacted the help line.

"The memory that remains most vivid is a phone call I got on the help line from someone who had evacuated from Fukushima. The person had evacuated on their own, not like Futaba where the whole town had to evacuate. The family got separated during the evacuation and managed to end up in Saitama and Tokyo, but the person was completely alone. They spent the whole time crying on the phone, telling me that they didn't know what to do, and that the family was constantly fighting. They were thinking that it would be better if they all just died. There were many people like that – many cases of people in very serious situations, hiding that they were from Fukushima and that sort of thing. Some of the people who evacuated to Saitama Prefecture committed suicide, and some attempted. Even though we knew that sort of thing must be happening quite often, we don't know how often. The fact that cases like that exist means that there are huge numbers of potentially suicidal people living in isolation, and I think caring for such people is going to be a big issue in the future."

This incident shows that even though there were a great many evacuees dealing with difficulties, many were unable to receive help, and more than that, there wasn't even a clear understanding of extent to which help was needed. The SSN and the team at Waseda University started preparing a large-scale questionnaire survey in collaboration with Futaba Town Office and the Disaster Relief Liaison Committee to get a clearer picture of the current situation.

4. Improving the information environment

Aiko began working at the evacuation center as a part of his company Information Environment Communications, but after meeting the SSN at the Super Arena and again working together at Kisai High School, he was asked if he wanted to work together in a more organized way, and he joined the SSN.

Aiko learned that when Futaba Town Office relocated as a whole to Kisai High School, they would need 58 computers in order to function properly, and he used social networks and his connections with his former employers to ask computer manufacturers for donations. His efforts resulted in 21 second-hand operators and other companies offering help, part of which came in the form of a donation from Taiwanese computer manufacturer ASUS. The evacuees at Kisai High School were living in 40 classrooms, the gymnasium, the martial arts gym, and the student's hall, and the donations made it possible to put at least one computer in each room, with bigger spaces having five computers. Moreover, a wireless LAN provided connectivity to the entire school, and it was installed due to the generosity of NTT. A computer research leader was assigned to conduct information searches for each room, and they attempted to pass on information to as many people as possible. In the summer, the JRCS donated a 37-inch television for each room, which made it even easier for people to get news and other information. By collaborating with companies and other organizations in this way, Aiko was able to reach his goal of improving the information environment.

5. Forging connections through distributing relief supplies

Nagata was involved in the procurement and distribution of relief supplies even before the evacuation center relocated to Kisai High School. When the Super Arena center was closed and evacuees were moving into municipal housing and private apartments, Nagata learned from the people he had met at the Super Arena that their new lodgings weren't sufficiently stocked with daily necessities, and that places that needed relief supplies weren't receiving them. He listened to all of the comments, prepared the supplies, and began delivering them to the people who needed them. Nagata was able to fully harness the network of connections he had built through his

How to Practice Social Care by Collaboration between several professionality   43

work to get a better understanding of where supplies were concentrated, and to secure the means and the personnel needed to distribute those supplies.

Meanwhile, as the people became more dispersed after leaving the evacuation center, the closely-knit communities that had formed around them began to break apart. Nagata realized that this was happening, and as he procured relief supplies and distributed them to the evacuees, he also began working to ensure that the evacuees and the relief workers could maintain the relationships they had built with each other.

Thus, as the evacuees were moving from large-scale centers to individual lodgings, the relief workers continued to work to grasp the changing needs of the evacuees and determine what form support should take. Kisai High School operated as an evacuation center for two years and nine months, from April 1, 2011 to December 27, 2013. It is known for having been the last evacuation center to close after the 2011 Tohoku earthquake.

VI. Support efforts outside of evacuation centers

The supporters did various activities in addition to their work at the Saitama Super Arena and Kisai High School. Aiko took over administrative duties at the SSN and since July 2011, he has handled the creation of meeting minutes and reports, grant applications and management, and disseminating information about relief efforts and about get-togethers being held throughout the prefecture.

1. Administrative support for friendship organizations and community cafés

Seven years have passed since the earthquake and nuclear accident, and at this point, there are around 40 friendship organizations and community cafés for evacuees in Saitama Prefecture. Since 2012, Aiko has lent a hand in the administration of Aozora-Aozora discussion group in Tokorozawa, the Disaster Friendship Café in Niiza, and the Connection Café in Kasukabe. These get-togethers are used to learn about the conditions evacuees are facing, and as a place for them to talk about the things they worry about on a regular basis.

Special events have also been held since life has begun to settle down for the evacuees and they built friendships with the people they met at the get-togethers. In the past, many have gathered to sing songs, go on outings in the neighborhood, and to take part in summer evening parties and cherry blossom viewing events. Meanwhile, medical teams have also taken part in the get-togethers, where they offer check-ups and give advice on staying healthy. Students from Waseda University have also participated. Aiko still takes new requests from evacuees and plans out new activities.

As previously mentioned, Nagata was responsible for procuring and distributing relief supplies at the evacuation centers, and he has also put in the effort to hold get-togethers and discussion events to ensure the evacuees and relief supporters can remain close. The catalyst for his participation was an evacuee trip planned in March 2012. Those who had evacuated from Fukushima Prefecture would go on a trip around the prefecture for the first time in the year since the disaster, and it was partly meant to help them renew old friendships. Some of the participants saw people they hadn't seen in the entire course of the year, and when Nagata saw the happiness in their faces, he realized afresh that people weren't getting the chance to get out of their new neighborhoods and had little opportunity to meet other evacuees scattered around Saitama and other prefectures. There was a need for interaction between evacuees that wasn't being met. In order to respond to that need, discussion forums and other get-togethers were being launched so evacuees could meet and interact with each other in their new neighborhood. However, Nagata knew that there would be administrative obstacles to overcome, e.g. finding venues and securing equipment, so he decided that he would begin offering administrative support for these events.

> "We started the get-togethers and discussion events to make sure people could maintain the relationships they had made while living at the evacuation centers," Nagata said. "The evacuees themselves also held their own parties and discussion groups, as did local elderly women in their new neighborhoods, and the second stage of our work started there, so we could support their efforts."

2. Publishing PR magazines to support the evacuees

Nagata has been holding Fuku-Tama Meetings since 2012 as a forum for leaders running the various groups spread around Saitama, as a means of connecting with other support groups and promoting exchange and support within that wide network. In addition, he has also put much effort into the Fuku-Tama Tayori, a newsletter meant to promote interaction between the evacuees scattered throughout the prefecture. The first issue was made to provide information on the Fukushima trip in March 2012, and it was distributed to participants on the bus on the way there. The next issue was published in April 2012, and it was used to share the comments of the evacuees who took the trip and were able to reunite with others. In addition to their comments, information was provided on discussion sessions and other get-togethers which began being held around Saitama, events being held in the coming month, and information on the distribution of relief supplies. The Fuku-Tama Tayori was well-received and was published almost monthly thereafter.

> "One reason I wanted to publish the Fuku-Tama Tayori was to help motivate everyone. Next was to provide info," Nagata said. "There are so many different

groups and meetings around Saitama, but if you think about how big Saitama is, you realize that in a way they are being held in only a few limited places. More than that, some people can't attend even if they want to because they don't have cars, or have a hospital appointment on the day, that sort of thing. My hope is that by passing on information about events being held in various locations and at various times, they can choose the times that work for them, and will be able to motivate themselves to come out and meet new people."

Even seven years after the disaster, information continues to be communicated to evacuees through the Fuku-Tama Tayori. It has helped evacuees connect with each other and has led to many reunions.

3. Holding supporter training courses

Hagiwara has provided support in her role as a clinical psychologist, and in addition to her work with evacuees, she has also been involved with providing training sessions targeted at relief workers. The 2012 Gatekeeper Training Course focused on roleplaying activities designed to give participants the fundamental listening skills necessary to interpersonal support. The Evacuee Support Organizers Course has been running since 2013, and that course offers workshops that show participants how to listen to people's problems and put them in touch with publicly-available resources such as legal help, social welfare, government contacts, and private support organizations.

"I have been working with a group of other clinical psychologists, and we conducted training in our role as the SSN mental health support team," Hagiwara said. "My experience teaching clinical psychology was helpful there. Up until now, I've always thought there's no point in having clinical psychologists on site if they aren't going to be offering medical care, but it was a great feeling to see how useful my own educational experience has been."

As shown above, these individuals have not only provided support at evacuation centers, but they engage in a variety of activities tailored to meet the changing needs in diverse areas.

VII. Post-operational reflections

All six individuals who participated in the support operations detailed here found the experience truly meaningful, and it seems that it will have a large influence on their future professional lives as well.

Inomata continues to work with victims as he has done since the disaster. When talking about the time before he joined the relief effort, he told us that he "gained a lot of things by participating in the support activities." One of those things was "an expanded network." Through the mutual efforts conducted at the Super Arena, Inomata met many people he had never met before, with different areas of expertise. He used those connections to start a new support effort called the Yorisoi Hotline. Yorisoi means "come together," and the hotline was launched in the three prefectures most affected by the disaster –Iwate, Miyagi, and Fukushima – in October 2011. It was then folded into the Cabinet Office in March 2012 and launched in Saitama and the rest of the country. The telephone help line accepts calls 24-hours-a-day for consultations on daily living, domestic violence and sexual assault, issues faced by sexual minorities, and more. It offers a means for callers to find the solutions they need by connecting them to legal, social welfare, and government help desks, and to private support organizations. Inomata was put in charge of the Yorisoi Hotline's Saitama center, and told us that his relief work post-disaster had a real effect on his work afterwards, with people he has met through the relief operations even taking part in the hotline.

> "I met many people while helping with the disaster relief efforts, and they taught me many things," Inomata said. "I think the experience helped me to expand the range of work I can do as a lawyer."

As previously mentioned, Hirose's goal was to find something he could do to help other people and society as a whole, and that led him to lending a hand in a variety of different support activities. He told us what the term "3.11" means to him, and what he got out of his work.

> "For me and many other people, I think 3.11 was a turning point, when we looked at ourselves and what 'society' means," Hirose explained. "It became the catalyst for people to think more deeply about the issues surrounding life and death. I think everyone began to think about their own lives thus far and about social movements as many people volunteered to help, everyone cut their electricity use, and opposition to the continued use of nuclear power surged. The disaster was a real tragedy, but it gave people the opportunity to think about various things, and I think it opened people's eyes to the fact that we can work together and help each other."

Hagiwara looked at the situation faced by those forced to evacuate from the earthquake damage and the nuclear accident, and took it head-on. As a professional, she felt helpless in the face of the sheer absurdity of the extent of the disaster. However, she was also moved by the people of Tohoku who had to eke out an existence in the most desperate of circumstances, and by the other experts who worked hard to do whatever they could to help.

"It was really the strength of the people of Tohoku," Hagiwara said. "They were able to keep it in the face of that insanity, and it made me realize just how strong humanity is. I also saw many people working themselves to exhaustion after the earthquake, people from all professions. That experience has become a source of inspiration for me in my life. That sense of connecting with the people of Tohoku and with the people who offered their help has made me a better person."

For Aiko, the events around the disaster helped him get a better understanding of what it means to be Japanese. More specifically, this realization came about after talking to a woman in her 60s from Soma who he met during his relief work.

"The story of a woman in her 60s who I met while setting up equipment for a meeting is really symbolic to me," Aiko said. "She said to me, 'The character for kizuna (bond) is made up of the characters for 'thread' and 'half,' right? Well, I really like the character *yui* (mutual help), because it's written using the characters for 'thread' and for 'luck.' According to that woman, the word kizuna is like a set of reins, symbolizing the relationship between a person and a horse, but yui symbolizes Fukushima in that it represents working together to help each other. When I heard that, I thought about how great a country Japan is. So, for me, 3.11 is when I learned about what lies at the heart of the Japanese people."

Takano experienced poverty first-hand before taking part in these support efforts, and he told us why he continued to support the evacuees since March 11, 2011.

"In a way, the evacuees have to fight a battle every day to live," Takano said. "They have to fight for many different things, not just to get compensation, but all the things they need to survive. When I joined this fight, it was because I decided that this is where I have to draw the line; if I broke here, I would be the one who lost. That's why I'm certain that I'll keep working with them into the future."

Takano's desire to stick by someone's side is apparent from the first time people meet him. The people who came for consultations were able to build relationships with him, resting assured that he would have their backs. For them, the fact that Takano stayed by their sides was in itself a big source of support. He told us that he still believes the relationships he makes with people he meets are very important, and he hopes he can work with them to help make society a place for people to live together.

Finally, Nagata told us that these support activities helped him build new relation-

48   Part I - 2

ships not only with people from Fukushima, but also with people already living in Saitama.

> "Of course, it would be better if people didn't have to live as evacuees," Nagata said, "but the disaster led to me meeting many people, and I'm really thankful for getting the chance to work with them. I learned about the delicious food you can get in Fukushima Prefecture, and they all brought in local Fukushima dishes that I had a chance to try. For me, it gave me a new life and new things to enjoy, and I think that was a good part of it."

In Nagata's words, we get a sense for how these efforts have shown that we have moved forward hand-in-hand, helping each other, with no hierarchy between those helping and those being helped.

VIII. General Discussion: The significance of multidisciplinary collaboration

In this chapter, we have discussed how six supporters formed teams of experts from different fields and conducted questionnaire surveys to uncover the changing needs of people after the earthquake and nuclear power plant accident, and how they have used those results to plan out relief work in an organized effort to provide victims of the disaster with the support they need. In addition, we discussed how these support activities have continued, with each individual always working hard to share information and work towards common objectives by making maximum use of each of their fields of expertise without it just ending up as a simple division of labor.

Based on his experiences in conducting relief efforts in the aftermath of the 1995 Kobe earthquake, Murakami (2006) argued that the pain disaster victims experience comes in different forms – physical, mental, social, and spiritual – and it is necessary to provide total human care through teams formed of people in different occupations. After the 2004 Chuetsu earthquake in Niigata Prefecture, a Hyogo Prefecture Mental Health Team established a mental health care clinic at a nursery school serving as an evacuation center in the Niigata city of Ojiya. It was staffed by individuals with different specialties who had experienced the Kobe earthquake, including experts in psychiatry, clinical nursing, public health nursing, clinical psychology, and psychiatric social work. Shunichiro Iwao was a doctor who worked with the Hyogo team, and Iwao (2007) describes how unexpected situations regularly arise when providing relief support in disaster areas, and that it is effective to "study (situations on site) from multiple perspectives offered by different specialized fields" and to make use of the "expanded networks" made possible through such participation. Regarding relief efforts after the 2011 Tohoku earthquake as well, there were numerous reports of the successes achieved by multidisciplinary relief teams (Hirano 2014; Yonekura 2018; Matsui 2018).

Multidisciplinary collaboration is also being recommended in international relief efforts as well. Mollica, R.F., et al. (2013) have worked around the world providing trauma care to displaced peoples in Cambodia, Croatia, Bosnia, and other disaster and conflict locations. From that experience, they have created methodologies bringing together clinical case studies, quantitative and qualitative research, epidemiology, oral life histories, literature, and more, and they have developed psychological and social care regimens for survivors of various types of society-level violence and torment. Mollica is Director of the Harvard Program in Refugee Trauma (HPRT), which is staffed by various specialists, including psychiatrists, social workers, community organizers, clinical psychologists, NGO experts, epidemiologists, neuroscientists, pediatricians, medical anthropologists, journalists, and theologians.

The importance of multidisciplinary collaborations is becoming clearer and clearer, not only in relief operations conducted during disasters, conflicts, and other emergencies, but also in various other support provided in more peaceful times, probably due to the perceived complexities of the different needs of individuals and groups requiring support.

Murata (2011) researches multidisciplinary health and welfare service collaborations between different specialist organizations. According to Murata, the needs of relief and support recipients are expanding and becoming more diverse in modern Japanese society, and there are limits to how well single occupations can respond to those comprehensive needs. Therefore, collaboration and cooperation between individuals in different fields are needed to successfully provide an appropriate response.

As this chapter has shown, by bringing together experts from multiple disciplines, it becomes possible to get a better understanding of victim needs and issues that are easily overlooked, and thereby determine what relief is most necessary from a diverse range of perspectives. This allows not only for the planning of short-term support operations, but also for the planning of long-term operations. In addition, a forum for information and opinion sharing is an essential part of making effective use of such a diverse range of expertise. During support operations conducted at Saitama Super Arena, Saitama prefecture's social welfare council took the lead to gather representatives of the SSN and other support groups for daily group leader meetings. As described by Iwao (2007), the face-to-face interactions allowed by the opinion exchange and information sharing between the various support groups were not simply to aid in the division of labor between people in different specialties. They allowed them to share a common goal, and thereby encouraged them to value the relationships they built with their colleagues and a sense of teamwork.

Next, another advantage of the multidisciplinary collaboration may have been the construction of the network by each expert. The group leader meetings conducted immediately after the disaster at Saitama Super Arena led to the extended networks of supporters that arose after the evacuation center was shut down. The needs of disaster victims changed as time passes, and it was thought that having networks made up of individuals in multiple areas of expertise would make it possible to respond flexibly to various situations and to continue providing support over the mid- to long-term. Based on the networking theory of Lipnack and Stamps, Kakegawa (2010) suggested that networks can be characterized in the following way: 1. They integrate their different parts into the whole; 2. each level of the network is important; 3. they are decentralized; 4. they are multifaceted; and 5. they have multiple leaders. The examples presented here confirm his theory. Uenoya, et al. (2013) describe the importance of using practical knowledge about disaster areas in the building of local communities thereafter under the concept of "disaster social work." This research also supports that theory, as the experience of engaging in multidisciplinary collaboration during times of disaster can potentially be applied to problem resolution in times of peace.

Finally, we have shown that multidisciplinary collaboration is not only an effective means of providing support; it helps professionals grow in their own field of expertise. We have clearly shown that, by working alongside people in other professional fields, one's own perspective is broadened at the same time as one is provided an opportunity to reconsider how to best provide support in one's role as a specialist.

Regarding the consultation services themselves, clinical psychologist Yuko Hagiwara said, "The atmosphere of stability and flexibility that the lawyers and judicial scriveners gave out when they were providing consultations to the evacuees left a big impression on me." Meanwhile, judicial scrivener Takashi Hirose said, "The way the clinical psychologists worked made me continuously think about what sort of care was needed and what sort of care could be provided." In this way, the multidisciplinary support efforts truly served as a forum for collaborative learning, as professionals from different fields of expertise worked closely together, each gaining much from the experience. That professional growth will not only expand their potential as individual support workers, but it will also expand the potential of multidisciplinary collaboration for the future.

IX. Conclusion

This chapter provided a glimpse into the practical side of the social care provided through multidisciplinary collaboration in Saitama after the 2011 Tohoku earthquake and nuclear power plant disaster. This was accomplished through the narratives of six individuals in different fields of expertise who are members of the Shinsai Shien Network Saitama (SSN), one partner of which is our Waseda University team. It illustrates how each of these supporters thought, acted, and collaborated in response to the constantly changing situation post-disaster. In addition, we also clearly show that these support efforts were deeply significant for each of the six individuals, and that their experiences could potentially contribute greatly to their future professional work.

Our survey, research, and support team is made up of educators, researchers, and students at Waseda University, and it was a very exciting experience for us to meet these individuals – a lawyer, a judicial scrivener, a clinical psychologist, a systems engineer, a social worker, and a specialist in labor welfare – and for our research to make a direct contribution to problem resolution in our society. We treasure having had this chance to collaborate – to have shared a common goal in responding to the disaster.

Multidisciplinary collaborations are not limited to times of disaster. We expect such collaborations will be used in the future to provide support to the financially disadvantaged, to support the ill and disabled, to render aid to immigrants, refugees, and minorities, and in various other support efforts.

References

Hirano, T., 2014. *Daishinsai to chiiki fukushi no kadai – 2010 nendai*. [Issues in large-scale earthquakes and community welfare – 2010s.], Hirano, T., Harada, M. (Ed.), *Chiiki fukushi no tenkai (Kaitei ban)*. [Development of Community Welfare (Revised Edition).], Hōsō daigaku kyōiku shinkō kai. [Foundation for the Promotion of the Open University of Japan.]

Iwao, S., Katsurayama, H., Mitsuchiro, N., et al., 2007. *Saigaiji no seishin hoken katsudō ni okeru tashokusyu renkei no igi: chūetsu daishinsaiji no hyōgo ken kokoro no kea chīmu no katsudō kara*. [Importance of multidisciplinary collaboration in mental health support in times of disaster: From the activities of the Hyōgo Prefecture Mental Health Care Team after the Chuetsu earthquake.], *The Japanese journal of hospital and community psychiatry*, 49 (3), 42-44.

Kakegawa, N., 2010. *Saigai to chiiki nettowāku*. [Disaster and Community Networks.], Nishio, Y., Otsuka, Y., Furukawa, T. (Ed.), 2010. *Saigai fukushi towa nanika; seikatsu shien taisei no kōchiku ni mukete*. [What is Disaster Welfare; Towards the construction of a social support system.], Minerva Shobō, pp. 93-106.

Lipnack, J., Stamps, J., 1982. Networking, the First Report and Directory. New York: Doubleday & Company, Inc., ISBN 0-385-7772-0 AACR2.

Matsui, S., 2018. *Hisaichi e hairi, renkei wo tsukuru*. [Entering the disaster area, creating cooperation.], Maeda, M. (Ed.), *Fukushima gempatsu jiko ga motarashita mono*. [What the Fukushima Nuclear Accident Brought About.], Seishin Shobō, pp.228-246.

Mayumi, M., 2011. A Basic Study on Interprofessional Collaboration in Health and Social Care; Code of Ethics for Health Care Professionals. *Otsuma Women's University bulletin of Faculty of Human Relations*, 13, 159-165.

Murakami, N., Ozasa, Y., Muramatsu, S., 2006. Psychosomatic Medicine in Disasters: Experiences of Psychosomatic Physician in the Hanshin-Awaji and Niigata-Chuetsu Earthquakes Disaster Areas. *Jpn J Psychosom Med*, 46, 655-660.

Mollica, R.F., 2013. Textbook of Global Mental Health: Trauma and Recovery, A Companion Guide for Field and Clinical Care of Traumatized People Worldwide. Harvard Program in Refugee Trauma, ISBN 9781257995899.

Tsujiuchi, T., Yamaguchi, M., Masuda, K., Tsuchida, M., Inomata, T., Kumano, H., Kikuchi, Y., Augusterfer, E.F., Mollica, R.F., 2016. High prevalence of post-traumatic stress symptoms in relation to social factors in affected population one year after the Fukushima nuclear disaster. *PLoS One*, 11(3), e0151807. doi:10.1371/journal.pone.0151807.

Uenoya, K. (Sup.Ed.), 2013. *Saigai sousharu wāku nyūmon; hisaichi no jissenchi kara manabu*. [Introduction to Disaster Social Work: Practical knowledge learned in the disaster area.], Chūō hōki Publishing Co., Ltd.

Yonekura, K., 2018. *Nagomi no katsudō kara; shinsai ni okeru kokoro no tasyokusyu chīmu no kiseki*. [The activities of Nagomi; Tracing mental health care in a disaster area provided by a multidisciplinary team.], Maeda, M. (Ed.), *Fukushima gempastu jiko ga motarashita mono.* [What the Fukushima Nuclear Accident Brought About.], Seishin Shobō, pp. 199-227.

3 Physical Health / Public Health / Policy Making

Supporting the public healthcare system after a disaster

Tamotsu Nakasa MD [1][2][5] *(Global Health and Medicine)*,
Ryo Sasaki [3], *Yasuo Sugiura* [2], *Yoichi Horikoshi* [2], *Jin Murakami* [2],
Keiko Ouchi [4], *Shinichiro Noda* [2], *Tomomi Kitamura* [2],
Hidechika Akashi [2]

Key words: coordination, health administration, subacute phase

Abstract

The Great East Japan Earthquake caused major damage to lifelines, healthcare facilities, and government organizations across an extensive area. The effects of the disaster were felt particularly strongly within the public healthcare system, which saw reduced numbers of administrative and medical personnel; halted distribution of medicines and other medical supplies; blackouts, water supply cutoffs, and loss of other infrastructure; poor use of mobile phones and other methods of communication to disseminate information; and an inability on the parts of the national and prefectural governments to provide appropriate guidance. Immediately after the disaster struck, the National Center for Global Health and Medicine began providing medical and administrative support to the area around the cities of Higashimatsushima and Ishinomaki, but direct medical support is not the only type of assistance needed after such an event. What is most important is to provide continuous support to the primary disaster response body in a region – the public health services – throughout the acute (immediately after the disaster strikes), sub-acute, and recovery phases.

---

[1] Visiting Professor, School of Tropical Medicine and Global Health, Nagasaki University
[2] International Medical Cooperation Department, National Center for Global Health and Medicine
[3] Emergency Department, National Center for Global Health and Medicine
[4] Health and Welfare section, City of Higashimatsushima
[5] Visiting Researcher, Waseda Institute of Medical Anthropology on Disaster Reconstruction (WIMA)

I. Introduction

The Great East Japan Earthquake struck on 11 March 2011 and caused great amounts of damage across a vast area (Fig. 1). Lifelines were cut, health and welfare infrastructure was damaged, and many government offices and organizations were destroyed. The effects of the disaster were felt particularly strongly within the public healthcare system, which saw reduced numbers of government and medical personnel due to the disaster; halted distribution of medicines and other medical supplies; blackouts, water supply cutoffs, and loss of other infrastructure; poor use of mobile phones and other methods of communication to disseminate information; and an inability on the parts of the national and prefectural governments to provide appropriate guidance. It was an extremely difficult situation for people used to public health services and medical care provided by sufficient personnel, material, money, and information, and was reminiscent of the healthcare system of a developing country.

• Extent of damage caused by the disaster	
	As of 27 December 2011
Number of remains recovered, number of dead and missing	
Recovered remains	1,046 individuals (As of 27 December 2011)
Deaths (Higashimatsushima residents)	1,002 individuals (As of 27 December 2011)
Missing (Not yet confirmed safe)	61 individuals (As of 27 December 2011)
Lifeline Damage/Loss	
Electricity disruptions (As of 29 July 2011)	22,574 homes (number of contracts) Restored 19,437 homes
Gas leaks	Unknown
Water cut (As of 20 December 2011)	15,012 homes (number of contracts) Restored 13,942 homes Unrestored 1,070 homes
Homes Damaged (As of 6 December 2011)	
Completely destroyed (including washed away by tsunami)	5,463 homes (1,266 washed away)
Mostly destroyed	3,046 homes
Partially destroyed	2,477 homes
Sub-total (Homes completely, mostly, or partially destroyed as ratio of total)	10,986 homes (72.7% of total)
Partially damaged	3,546 homes
Total (Overall Ratio)	14,532 homes (96.1% of total)
Road damage	
In city limits	Unknown

Figure 1. Extent of damage in city of Higashimatsushima

Immediately after the disaster struck, the National Center for Global Health and Medicine (NCGM) dispatched a DMAT to the Tohoku region in response to this catastrophe and it operated primarily in the area around the cities of Higashimatsushima and Ishinomaki in Miyagi Prefecture. Subsequently, NCGM also deployed continuously medical teams to patrol evacuation centers operated by the city of Higashimatsushima, and public hygiene teams to help support and maintain public health (Fig. 2). The teams treated more than 1,000 patients and supported surveys on the health of disaster victims still living in their own homes, and beginning in July of that year, NCGM entered into a one-year support agreement with Higashimatsushima to undertake efforts in support of public healthcare services. This paper serves as a report of those activities.

II. Public healthcare support requirements

This disaster was unique because of the sheer amount of damage caused to many public healthcare facilities, including health centers and social welfare centers, and because many public health employees were also victims. This resulted in the public health system itself failing to function properly, and it became necessary to provide support for that system. In addition, it is said this earthquake resulted in a lower ratio of serious injuries to deaths than might be expected in a normal earthquake due to

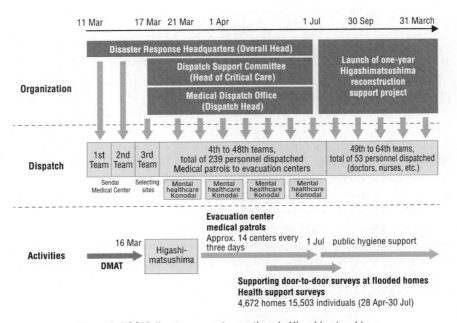

Figure 2. NCGM disaster support operations in Higashimatsushima

the subsequent tsunami. The numbers support this theory, with the total number of deaths standing at 15,843 – 92.5% due to drowning, 4.4% due to traumatic injury, and 1.1% from injuries due to fire (data from National Police Agency announcement made in December 2011.) There were few seriously injured individuals to treat and adequate medical treatment was provided at major hospitals, as they had the support of DMATs immediately after the disaster. In those conditions, patients in the disaster area were primarily made up of large numbers of lightly-injured and elderly disaster victims. Medical statistics were gathered during evacuation center patrols conducted between 22 March and 10 May in the Higashimatsushima area NCGM had taken responsibility for. The data shows that in the cold weather directly after the disaster, the majority of patients were those seeking treatment of upper respiratory tract infections such as common colds, and those suffering from allergic rhinitis, thought to be caused by rubble dust and pollen. As temperatures rose more than a month later, there was a sharp decrease in upper respiratory tract infections, but there was an increase in the fraction of patients suffering from high blood pressure, insomnia and other ailments arising from post-disaster stress and issues connected to living long-term in evacuation centers. In addition, there were issues in providing treatment to the elderly as 65% of those treated were aged 60 years or older.

Primary requirements after the disaster involved assessing initial conditions and setting up, operating, and managing evacuation centers that could provide medical treatment. Public health department staff were responsible for these actions, and the efforts were primarily handled by public health nurses, who were incredibly busy both operating the evacuation centers and providing care to individual victims. After the disaster, these public health officials ended up staying at the health centers and government offices, and the volume of work they were doing was well beyond their capacity – help was needed. Evacuation center management requires public health officials, and particularly public health nurses, to perform an enormous and diverse array of duties, including securing and maintaining electricity, water, and toilets to improve the living environment, managing influenza and other infectious diseases, and providing mental health care to victims. They also had to provide orientation to medical support teams deployed at short intervals of between three and seven days, and had to coordinate medical treatment and work assignments as well. Even though they appreciated the outside assistance being offered, they had to listen to the varied and numerous opinions of those providing support and found it very difficult to respond to their requests. Immediately after the disaster, support was essential. What is needed in such a framework are experts with knowledge of public healthcare system, hygiene management, and disaster medicine who can play a supporting role for public health officials. Also needed is an approach through which support can be offered.

During the sub-acute phase, it is necessary to assess various requirements in addition

Supporting the public healthcare system after a disaster   59

to managing the above-mentioned evacuation centers and coordinating the efforts of the different support teams on the ground. Assessments must be conducted after a disaster to allow for better response to the daily changing needs of evacuation centers, to determine the needs of a region as a whole, and to provide the necessary relief to those unable able to obtain support. This work is administered by government agencies. One particularly necessary duty is the implementation of home visits to determine the needs of disaster victims living in homes that suffered comparatively little damage. This type of health support survey was conducted in Higashimatsushima as well, beginning in late April.

During the recovery phase, there was increased necessity to resume conducting postpartum examinations, maternity checkups, infant checkups, vaccinations and other such activities that had been halted. In fact, such activities were resumed in Higashimatsushima over the May holidays, two months after the disaster. In June, temporary housing having been built, medical operations at evacuation centers were brought to an end and many people had moved into the temporary housing by July and August. However, it was expected that a number of issues would arise in that sudden change from communal living to individual living, with evacuees having to deal with loneliness and the financial burden of obtaining food and other items, so support was deemed necessary. In addition, with the decrease in available external support, there was a gradually increasing dissatisfaction regarding the unequal support being offered to those living at home, so a response to that issue was also determined to be necessary.

III. Supporting relief coordination

There was an immense and varied outpouring of support from all around the country after the disaster, but there were issues in how to coordinate the various support teams, each of which would stay in the disaster area for a relatively short time. Coordination efforts suffered, and there were problems with teams being unable to complete the work they originally set out to do. Rather than having clinical medicine/health care personnel coordinate efforts like these, it is more appropriate to assign such work to public health nurses with experience in public health administration, and to other individuals with a better overall understanding of public hygiene. These types of personnel can be expected to build more effective collaborative relationships with coordinators within public health administrative bodies. In addition, since those providing support are fundamentally only active temporarily and the primary actors who will be running such operations are people from the affected region, external support must be designed to aid regional facilities in restoring their ability to operate independently.

As illustrated in Fig. 3, the response to this disaster made more effective by installing lead public health nurses as government coordinators, then having the external supporters (NCGM Bureau of International Health Cooperation personnel with experience in supporting national-level public healthcare administration) work behind the scenes supporting management efforts (Figs. 3, 4). In more concrete terms, personnel participated in regional coordination meetings, helped draw up medical team treatment outreach programs, provided orientations for external medical teams, provided various planning support, and aided in data entry and analysis of assessments and health surveys.

IV. Supporting at-home living (Health support surveys)

After the disaster, Higashimatsushima reported that 65% of the city had been flooded and damaged. Many people stayed home in houses that weren't washed away but had suffered damage to their ground floors. Immediately after the disaster, support was primarily being offered to those who had completely lost their homes and evacuated to shelters, and medical patrols were also primarily focused on providing treatment at evacuation centers.

In reality, many of those who stayed home in houses that weren't washed away did so out of respect for those whose homes had been swept away, and because they were

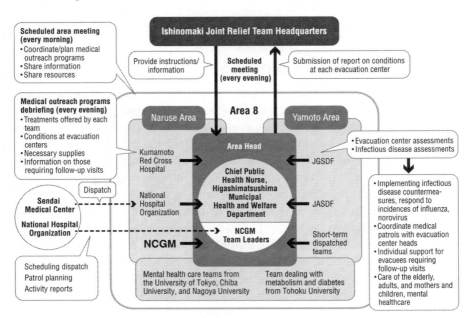

Figure 3. Outline of support activities by public health category

not at evacuation centers, they were unable to obtain information, food, and other forms of support, and it was reported that conditions continued to deteriorate for them. In order to get a better understand of the medical needs of those still living in their homes, health support surveys began to be conducted door-to-door a month and a half after the disaster in areas that had suffered flooding but had not been completely swept away by the tsunami.

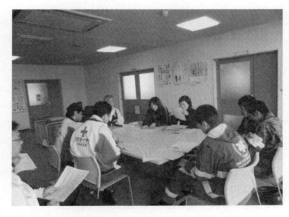

Figure 4. Supporting public health nurses

Surveys were conducted in pairs made up of public health nurses, hospital nurses and other health care workers. They visited damaged homes, interviewed all of the inhabitants, and measured blood pressures. During the interviews, they were asked about conditions after the disaster and if anyone was suffering from chronic illnesses. They had their blood pressure checked taken, were asked about any issues with coughing, and were asked other questions to help determine if they were suffering from any psychological or other abnormal issues (Table 1).

Table 1. Health support survey items

Address (Copied from Basic Resident Register)
1. Sources of information
2. Name
3. Have chronic disease? (current medical history)
4. Blood pressure
5. Have persistent cough?
6. Aware of own health?
7. Current mental state (5 items to screen for depression and PTSD)
8. Living conditions
9. Notes
10. Follow-up info (Necessary or not, request medical team or public health nurse intervention)
11-1. Living environment, habits (Damage/flooding conditions of house, access to lifelines) 11-2. Changes in diet/habits and exposure to seawater (in previous two weeks)

The surveys were conducted over the course of three months between 28 April and 28 July. They were completed at 4,672 of the 6,500 homes targeted and covered a total of 15,503 respondents.

The objective was to identify those requiring urgent care due to aggravated chronic illnesses, hypertension, or mental issues among disaster victims living in homes, and offer them the services they needed. An additional goal was to determine the needs of inhabitants. The surveys identified individuals in need of psychological treatment, and by obtaining blood pressure data for more than 4,000 people, the surveys also highlighted that there had been a significant increase in the number of people who had not taken hypertension medicine before the disaster, but had seen a spike in blood pressures subsequent to the disaster.

V. Public hygiene activities

1. Evacuation center nutrition surveys
Experience in previous large-scale disasters showed that nutrition intake at evacuation centers tends to be lower than desired. Periodic surveys were conducted to ensure evacuees were obtaining appropriate levels of nutrition. Results of the nutrition surveys conducted by nutritionists in Higashimatsushima can be found in Table 2, and the data shows that nutrition gradually increased from the 1,400-kilocalorie intake confirmed during the first survey.

2. Preventing food poisoning
With the arrival of summer, there were concerns about the occurrence of food poisoning arising from improper handling of bento boxes and poor hygiene management in kitchens. So, efforts to prevent food poisoning were begun when infectious disease countermeasures were implemented in July. Efforts were handled by on-site patrols comprised of one nutritionist from the health promotion department and one to two public health nurses who conducted interviews and inspections regarding bento

Table 2. Nutrition Survey (Higashimatsushima)

	Energy (kcal)	Protein (g)	Vitamin B1	Vitamin B2	Vitamin C
Survey 4, 20 July	2,033 kcal	64.0 g	0.81 mg	1.03 mg	57.3 mg
Survey 3, 2 June	2,045.6 kcal	72.8 g	1.4 mg	1.4 mg	19.3 mg
Survey 2, 20 May	1,642.2 kcal	59.2 g	0.7 mg	1.0 mg	50.0 mg
Survey 1, 8 April	1,396.8 kcal	47.1 g			
Nutrition Targets (After revision)	1,800-2,200 kcal	55.0 g or more	0.9 mg or more	1.0 mg or more	80.0 mg or more

handling and kitchen food hygiene. They provided guidance on the spot, hung posters providing information on bento box handling (storage and disposal), distributed pamphlets, provided information to representatives, distributed pamphlets on hygiene management during food preparation, provided guidance to representatives, provided information on food handling, confirmed that external supporters providing food were following hygienic practices, etc.

3. Health care for mothers and children

One month after the earthquake, requests for health care services for mothers and children (which had also been halted in Higashimatsushima since the disaster) began to arrive from the citizens who were not a victim, and it became necessary to resume those services. Beginning in late April, postpartum examinations, infant vaccinations, 4-month, 18-month and 3-year-old growth monitoring and other services were restored with outside assistance. The Japanese Midwives Association offered its support in offering post-partum examinations from late April, and vaccination and growth monitoring services were resumed by local physicians who had recovered from the disaster, and by pediatricians dispatched by NCGM.

VI. Public healthcare support after medical operations ended at evacuation centers

With the completion of temporary housing between June and July in Higashimatsushima, evacuees living at evacuation centers rapidly began moving in. Evacuation center management operations had been brought to an end, but it then became impor-

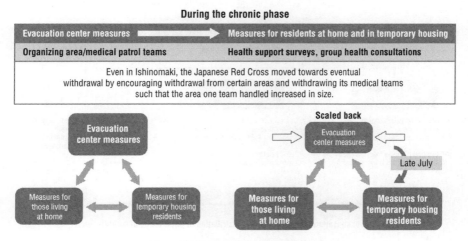

Figure 5. Time periods of the disaster

tant to answer the needs of those living at home and in temporary housing (Fig. 5).

In cooperation with the city of Higashimatsushima, it was decided that NCGM would support these public health efforts, and a one-year agreement to that effect was signed with the city. The agreement essentially stated that the city of Higashimatsushima had suffered major damage during the Great East Japan Earthquake and subsequent tsunami, and in order to restore public health and sanitation in the city, the city would work in collaboration with NCGM. NCGM would support the efforts by: conducting surveys on resident living environments and health conditions; supporting measures aimed at restoring public health and hygiene operations; offering personal public health services to the greatest extent possible; and providing advice and recommendations on other overall public health and hygiene administrative issues. For the municipal government, which had received a large amount of assistance in the short term, there were three benefits to having a single institution promise long-term support: 1) there was no longer any need to look for new sources of support; 2) there was no need to explain the situation to newcomers repeatedly; and 3) it became possible to receive continuous, strategically implemented assistance. Public healthcare support has been offered for two to three days a week since then as

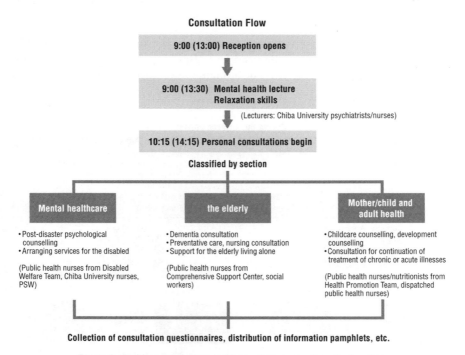

Figure 6. Health consultation meetings at temporary housing locations

at March 2012.

People in Higashimatsushima gradually began to move into temporary housing in May, and 25 locations offering 1,753 residences had been completed by August. People had awaited the chance to move out of the communal, low-privacy living environments of the evacuation centers, but the former evacuees were being forced from the large groups of the evacuation centers where all food, clothing and shelter was supplied, to living alone or with family in completely new living environments. For this reason, it was decided that public health measures had to be implemented for those living in temporary housing. First, health consultations began to be offered for the residents, then surveys were conducted at all temporary housing locations. Assistance was also provided for dental and oral health services, group rehabilitation guidance was offered, and health awareness activities were implemented (Fig. 6).

From 1 July to 21 October, a total of 20 health consultation meetings were held. Self-care counselling to help people deal with stress was provided at 17 of those meetings through the cooperation of Chiba University. A total of 244 people participated. Many of the participants were women, 30% were in their 60s, and half in their 70s or older. The most common reasons people participated were, in order: 1) to have blood pressure measured; 2) to ask for help dealing with insomnia and other mental issues; 3) to discuss physical condition; and 4) to ask about forgetfulness. Staff specialists responded to participant questions. Follow-ups were deemed necessary for 42 participants, and consultations were provided for 24 disabled individuals (insomnia, PTSD and other mental issues), 14 elderly individuals (forgetfulness, etc.), 5 adults

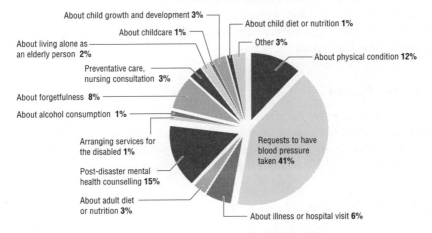

Figure 7. Health consultation participants (Total 244 individuals)

(interrupted treatments, domestic violence counselling, etc.) and zero mothers with children (Fig. 7).

The health support surveys provided a better understanding of conditions among victims living at home, but those victims inevitably received reduced levels of support when compared to those living in temporary housing (who were the subject of much more attention and thereby more support). This led to a rise in requests for help from these "at-home victims", who had until that point not expressed their dissatisfaction with the situation because they had been fortunate enough to still have homes. Health consultation meetings were begun in September to get a better grasp on the mental and physical health issues faced by those living in their original homes and to provide them with individualized support. Initial efforts involved measuring people's blood pressure and providing health consultations that gave people the chance to think about their own bodies and lifestyles through events such as the Tokyo Ota-ku Volunteer Group Lunch Exchanges and Nobiru Reconstruction Festival. Beginning in December, health workshops were provided for the at-home residents at each civic center.

Other measures were implemented to deal with the important issue of mental healthcare. Providing mental healthcare to victims of a disaster requires a support framework that allows for an understanding of the post-disaster transition in psychological state, the changing needs and required responses to those transitions, the state of available support resources, and the changing psychological conditions of those offering support to the resident victims, who had also been affected by the disaster. The University of Tokyo, Nagoya University, and Chiba University all cooperated in providing organizational support. In addition, mental healthcare was divided into four categories – child, adult, suicide countermeasures, and personnel – and operations were conducted in conjunction with evacuation center medical patrols and temporary housing support efforts.

VII. Conclusion

On 11 March 2012, a year has passed since the disaster, and the Tohoku region is still faced with very difficult conditions. However, public health officials are continuing to put their best efforts into rebuilding the system to allow for sustained and independent operation. They still need support to reach their goals.

References

Akashi, H., Miyoshi, C., Nakasa, T., et al., 2011. *Kokusai hoken iryō kyōryoku no keiken kara higashi nihon daishinsai shien wo kangaeru*. [Considering support offered after the Great East Japan Earthquake from experiences in international health and medical collaboration.], *Japan Medical Journal*, 4544, 28-31.

Sphere Project: Humanitarian Charter Humanitarian Response. 2011 Edition, 2011. Available from: http://www.sphereproject.org

The Code of Conduct for the International Red Cross and Red Crescent Movement and NGOs in Disaster Relief. Annex VI to the resolutions of the 26th International Conference of the Red Cross and Red Crescent, Geneva. 1995. Available from: http://www.ifrc.org/Docs/idrl/I259EN.pdf

---

* This chapter is based on the following paper: Nakasa, T., et al., 2012. Support for post-disaster health administration. *Japanese Journal of Disaster Medicine*, 17, 207-213.

4 Mental Health / Family Health / Community Health

Case study on support for voluntary evacuee families

From records of social gatherings aimed at children

Ryuhei Mochida MA[*1] *(Developmental psychology),*
Yuko Shiraishi MA[*2] *(Developmental psychology)*

Key words: voluntary evacuation, family support, children, empowerment

I. Introduction

The accident at Tokyo Electric Power Company's Fukushima Daiichi Nuclear Power Plant resulted in the evacuation of a great many people. The evacuees were forced to react instantly as they were torn from the lands they knew, compromising the relationships they had built and maintained for years with family, friends, and neighbors; as they searched for places to live and work, and faced many difficulties in the communities to which they evacuated. There were cases in which families themselves were forced apart, potentially forcing for the victims to reconsider the meaning of family itself.

We launched the *Kasasagi* Project in June of 2011 at the Developmental Ethology Laboratory at Waseda University's Graduate School of Human Sciences with the objective of supporting and studying families that evacuated to the Kanto area. Though on a smaller scale, we are still working on the project now in 2015 with a focus on Saitama Prefecture.

---

*1 Visiting Researcher, Advanced Research Center for Human Sciences, Waseda University
*2 Research Fellow, Center for Brain Science, Institute of Physical and Chemical Research (RIKEN)

70   Part I - 4

In this chapter, we would like to look a little closer at one of the many diverse activities undertaken as part of the *Kasasagi* Project[1], namely the support offered to children and guardians in families that found it difficult to adapt to their communities after evacuating to Saitama.

II. Evacuee support in Saitama Prefecture

Saitama Prefecture has more evacuees than most other places in the country (at 5,623 as of October 2015 according to the Saitama Prefecture website). According to Harada and Nishikido (2015), support in Saitama was characterized as being sought from municipalities and the private sector because, except for initially, the prefectural government offered only passive support to evacuees. Support can be broadly described as belonging to one of four categories, with necessary support periodically added (Table 1).

Here we will focus on the social gatherings In each community housing evacuees, social gatherings were held to provide a place for evacuees to meet and build relationships with other evacuees and with local volunteers. It is not easy to describe these social gatherings in a single phrase as the principles, scale, frequency, activities, and characteristics of participants were all dependent on the organization holding the gathering. However, gatherings presided over by support groups and evacuees themselves were held actively, and by August 2015, the number of groups had risen to more than 30.

---

1) *Kasasagi* (magpie) is a bird that bridges the stars Kengyuu (Altair) and Syokujyo (Vega), which are separated by the Milky Way, in a legend related to the Tanabata Festival known as the seasonal star festival in China, Japan, and some other Asian countries. The bird is a symbol of our project that aims link families separated by evacuation.

Case study on support for voluntary evacuee families   71

Table 1. Evacuee support in Saitama Prefecture

(This table is created by authors based on the report by Harada and Nishikido (2015))

	Support Type	Period	Details	Objective
1	Livelihood security through housing, supplies, legal counseling	From March 2011	Establishment of evacuation centers, introduction of housing provision/ borrowing system, reduction in/ exemption from water/sewerage fees (some municipalities only) distribution of home appliances, legal counseling, etc.	Help evacuees secure a livelihood
2	Holding of social gatherings	From April 2011	More than 30 organizations active as of September 2015, voluntary social gatherings of evacuees at housing complexes, social gatherings held for evacuees scattered across a wide area	Prevent isolation, help connect evacuees with local municipalities and support groups
3	Information sharing (Information magazines for evacuees)	From April 2012	Publication of Fukutama Dayori, as an information magazine for evacuees (4,000 published as of September 2015)	Provide information on social gatherings and other events to evacuees with difficulties obtaining information from the government, provide information on childcare, education, and health, collaborate between related groups, promote activities in other areas and encourage participation, etc.
4	Door-to-door visits by government/ private sector collaborations	From October 2011	Temporary city workers* and reconstruction assistants visiting evacuees in their residences, information sharing by municipal employees, professional organizations, private support groups and others providing support (the Disaster Liaison Council), meetings among relevant organizations, support groups, Fukushima Prefectural employees, the town office employees of four town in Futaba, (Fukutama Kaigi), meetings among relevant representatives (Fukutama Leader Kaigi)	Understand the needs of evacuees unable to attend social gatherings and connect them with specialist facilities

* Evacuees in the city were employed as temporary workers (From October 2011 in Koshigaya)

1. Social Gatherings as Self-Help Groups

We carried out a survey into the social gatherings held in Saitama Prefecture, and learned that participants included evacuees who formerly lived in what had become the designated evacuation zones of Fukushima Prefecture, evacuees from outside the designated evacuation areas, and those who had fled the destruction wrought by the tsunami. Many of the participants were in their 60s, and regardless of when the sessions were held, they primarily took the form of "salon cafés" and information sharing sessions (Mochida, 2012). During the gatherings, participants are able to meet up with others who lived in the same area or close to the same area before the earthquake, and they spend hours together, sharing memories, talking about how they have been doing recently, and discussing the problems they share.

In this way, these gatherings have become reminiscent of a sort of self-help group, providing people who share problems and goals in the same situation a place to spend time together communicating with each other. For a definition of self-help group, in this chapter, we reference Noguchi (2005) and Ito (2009), who defined such gatherings as "providing a means through which people in the same situation and sharing problems and goals can work together to find a way to resolve the issues they face through communication." Gartner and Riessman (1977/1985) presented the following six items as characteristic features of self-help groups: (1) The group always features relationships that are interactive and mutually influencing; (2) the group is always voluntary; (3) individual participation is important, and bureaucratization is not helpful (a more egalitarian approach is desired); (4) participants agree with and engage in the activities; (5) in many cases, the group has absolutely no power when first launched; (6) the group fulfills a need for a group that offers support (serving as a place to associate and identify with others, a hub of activities, a source of self-reinforcement (to realize one's own self.)) These descriptions are applicable to many evacuee social gatherings. However, taking the examples of the gatherings held in Saitama Prefecture, in addition to various other volunteers, they were also attended by legal professionals, clinical psychologists, and other specialists, so as self-help groups, the gatherings have taken a somewhat distinctive form.

Looking at the social gatherings from the self-help group perspective, the fact that participants are evacuees from a nuclear power plant accident may cause specific issues to arise. A number of opinions were offered during an interview survey conducted by the *Kasasagi* Project, namely that factions can form around people's place of origin and they can come into conflict; disagreements and struggles over members have arisen among the many participants; and families experiencing financial difficulties find it difficult to continue to attend social gatherings that require fees for registration or participation. The survey also uncovered the existence of a gap between needs and services offered, with survey respondents noting that what people are looking to obtain from the gatherings depends on the evacuees in question, and the difference between supporter intent and participant requirements. Other responses were more compelling: no matter where they go they are being told to "remain positive"; it is difficult to bring up more painful emotions; the pep talks they receive feel burdensome; and they worry about giving up before they get a chance to get in touch with those providing support (Hirata, et al., 2013). All are being labelled with the term "evacuee," but the situation they all find themselves in differs based on where they evacuated from and the level of damage done. When they are handled as a single homogenous group, the participants themselves feel the differences between themselves and other participants resulting in reactions like those above. This point will be discussed again later keeping in mind the example of social gatherings we held.

Tsujiuchi (2012) conducted a questionnaire survey of 2011 households that evacuated to Saitama Prefecture from Fukushima Prefecture (490 respondents/ 24.4% response rate). According to that survey, 20% of evacuees in Saitama answered that they had participated in a social gathering. The same survey conducted two years later (Tsujiuchi and Masuda, 2014) found that 29% of evacuees answered that they had participated in social gatherings. In addition, looking at the answers regarding overall importance of and level of satisfaction with the gatherings, they seemed to have been received well to a certain degree (Fig.1, Fig.2), showing that many evacuees find such events to beimportant.

Beginning in October 2012, we attended a number of gatherings in Saitama Prefecture, and noticed that not many children were participating. At that time, these social gatherings were essentially meant to be places for adults to meet, and there were essentially no gatherings designed for children to play the leading role. (Evacuee parents and children were invited to many other events during which they visited a theater or took some other type of excursion.)

There was meaning behind placing the focus of these gatherings on adult participants. The interview studies that we conducted, however, suggested that there may be children who have not yet become used to the communities to which they evacuated and need support. However, we had no access to such children, and felt that sufficient support for such children was unavailable. From that, we began thinking about how we could utilize our specialty to help, and decided to launch a social gathering aimed at children. However, it may be difficult to view such gatherings as a form of the self-help group evacuee social gatherings described thus far.

Beginning in the next section, we describe the puppet show program we ran in Saitama Prefecture, and discuss the significance of the social gatherings aimed at children as exemplified by the evacuee families who participated.

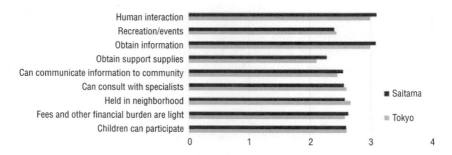

Figure 1. Important elements of community activities and social gatherings

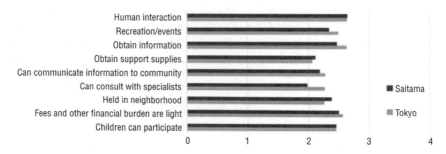

Figure 2. Current level of satisfaction with social gatherings and community activities

III. Evacuee family connecting with local communities through the puppet show program

In this section, we look at the activities conducted in the three years since we launched our program, with a focus on the evacuee families who participated in our gatherings. The content below is comprised of data gathered through interviews with guardians, video taken during activities, children's written impressions, notes taken during activities, and meeting records.

1. The Reasons for Puppet Shows

The puppet show format was adopted because puppet shows are appropriate for children, and they can get independently involved in the continued production and performance of such works. Because the puppet show "stage" hides the body of the performer, introverted or timid children can also easily take part. In addition, in holding the puppets, the performers can reconsider how to express various emotions and review physical actions and the forms of people and things (Matsuzaki, 2008). Also, the annual puppet show event allows them to set themselves a clear goal of taking part in the performance, which gives them a shared consciousness and future

Case study on support for voluntary evacuee families   75

activities to engage in as a group. The puppet show program involves a series of activities that includes story writing, puppet making, rehearsals, performances, and reflection meeting. In addition, there are two objectives behind the creation of puppet shows.

(1) Help evacuee families build interpersonal networks in their new communities
(2) Observe and support child development

The first objective in positioning puppet shows as a form of social gathering was to offer children an opportunity to form interpersonal relationships in the communities to which they evacuated, and bring together parental guardians raising children in unfamiliar communities with those already raising children in those communities. Puppet shows allow numerous performers to participate simultaneously, and through the process participants share time together with creating puppets, discussing content, and rehearsals, all of which are in line with the objectives as stated. In addition, while the children are rehearsing, parents and guardians can interact with each other. To achieve the objectives, little focus is placed on differences in the situations participants have found themselves in, no questions are asked about where they lived before evacuating or why they evacuated, and we actively invite families from the program's base in Tokorozawa City and the surrounding area, which sets the program apart from other evacuee social gatherings. In addition, with the children's development observed, DVDs of them in the program were sent to individuals who had lived with them before the earthquake (i.e. grandparents) thereby serving a psychological purpose, and when necessary, we also asked clinical psychologists and judicial scriveners to take part. As specialist knowledge and skills are needed to guide the creation of a puppet show, the shows were arranged with the cooperation of an NPO called Nouiku Network, which has been involved in helping elementary school students produce puppet shows for many years. They also provided guidance on the management of the shows, and due to our shared desire to support the evacuee families, the second and third programs were run as a collaboration between two groups. Moreover, undergraduate students in our laboratory also volunteered to take part.

2. Evacuee families that participated in the puppet show program

We used several methods to find participants for the program, including advertising in the Fukushima Dayori and local newspapers, and on local radio stations and our research group's website. We did not receive as many responses as expected. After some time, we noticed that many families were working through some difficult issues, with some having yet to decide whether they would remain in the new area, some having had to move multiple times, etc. Some evacuee children had to return to their homes in Fukushima each weekend because their relatives were there. In addition, some families were afraid to tell others that they were from Fukushima because they were worried about teasing and bullying. We were about to give up when we received a letter from the pseudonymously-named Matsui family, and they became the only evacuee family to take part in the puppet show program.

We provide some background on their situation. The family name Matsui and given names provided below were used to protect the family's privacy. Other details have been changed to ensure no hindrance lies in the way of discussing the family's situation.

A) Family composition
The Matsui family is a family of six that evacuated from Minamisoma to the suburbs of Tokorozawa. The family is made up of Yasuo (father, in his 40s), Saki (mother, in her 30s), Eiji (son, 10th grade), Masato (son, 8th grade), and Hana and Yuki (daughters, both 4th grade). (Ages and grades correspond to when the puppet show program began.) Before they evacuated, they lived with the paternal grandparents, but the grandparents were left behind in Minamisoma when they evacuated. Masato has been diagnosed with autism, and is taking special needs classes.

B) Participation in the puppet show program
The Matsui family had taken part in social gatherings for evacuees held near their homes post-evacuation, had received material support, and had been invited to dinner events, but had begun finding it more difficult to participate. Mother S explained the reason for that saying, "Even when we went, we were just treated like visitors," and that they had little time to interact with other families taking part. During that gathering, it seems that there was little opportunity for children to act on their own initiative, and that S also had difficulties herself in building relationships with others. This is why they became interested in the puppet show program, because it involved local families coming together regularly and practicing together towards a shared goal.

3. The Puppet Show Program and the Matsui Family
Here we take a look at some anecdotes regarding objectives (1) and (2) mentioned previously, and reflect on the puppet show program chronologically from beginning to end (see Fig.3). Quotation marks denote statements included as spoken.

A) Puppet Show Program 1 (November 2012 to August 2013)
Program 1 was the period during which the participants built relationships with each other, with the Matsui family and other local families coming together to share opinions and coordinate with puppet show staff, and to continue the activity. While only four families took part, the program was established and remained steadily active.

The goal was to hold a puppet show festival, and the performers put on a magnificent show, highlighting that the families and staff members seemed to have connected. While meetings continued to go well, one event shone the light on the difference in perspectives between the participants.

It occurred when participants selected the food for a barbecue meant to offer them a chance to reflect on the program. The Matsui family felt that, "anything from stores is fine," seemingly without any concern about where the food was from or about radiation. They had evacuated voluntarily, and to the parents, they felt much more secure in their new home in Tokorozawa than they would have in their old home at least. Food was another aspect in that anything grown in the area would be safer than items grown in the disaster area. However, one local family was concerned about the internal effects of exposure from food on their children, and they chose ingredients from shops with stricter standards than those set by the national government and ingredients from other countries.

In a later interview, Saki said, "If I was worried about what they're selling in supermarkets here, I'd never be able to return to Minamisoma. I'd never be able to go home." After hearing this, we thought that perhaps that difference in thinking regarding radiation and safety may have created a barrier in the relationship between the Mastui family and the other families that would extend beyond the forum of the puppet show. However, Mother Saki also said, "Just because we think differently doesn't mean we can't be friends."

This anecdote taught us that when considering what form support should take, we must also consider the significance of bringing together people of different viewpoints at social gatherings.

B) Puppet Show Program 2 (April 2014 to September 2014)
Nouiku Network, the organization that had provided guidance in running the puppet show, begin presiding over the puppet show for Progam2. Matsui daughters Hana and Yuki formed a new theater company with the aim of performing a puppet show at an event. They were unable to take part in the puppet show festival in Ikebukuro they participated in the previous year, but instead, they performed at the Iida Puppet Show Festival in Iida, Nagano Prefecture. The trip involved a stay of three nights and four days, but they had no worries about being separated from their parents and put on an excellent show.

Perhaps the children found it meaningful that they had not only performed a puppet show, but also travelled to various places and met many different people. By the time Program 2 had ended, the children had managed to make friends at school, and we felt that the puppet show program had fulfilled its role of helping the children build new relationships in the community to which they had evacuated. However, the children were enthusiastic about continuing, which led to the launch of Program 3.

C) Puppet Show Program 3 (September 2014 to September 2015)
By Program 3, the Matsui children had already had two years of experience in creating puppet shows, could consider the meaning of the shows for themselves, and they showed a stronger independence in taking part. The Matsui family, the staff, and the other members of the puppet show program shared time together for three years, and it seems that during that time their relationship became one of equals – a relationship that could no longer be appropriately described as one of "supporters and victims." The puppet show program was essentially run by children, and various perspectives were offered, and therefore some issues arose. We also could see that it allowed participation in the program to take various forms.

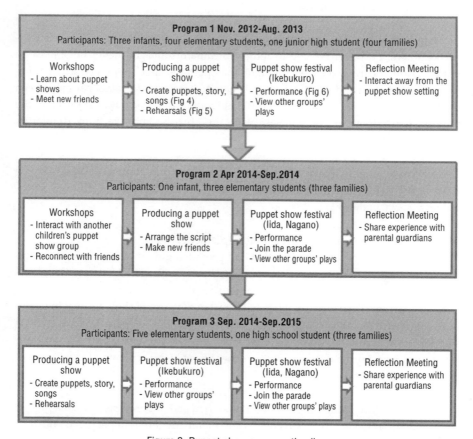

Figure 3. Puppet show program timeline

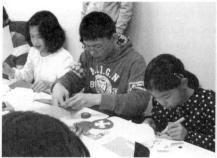
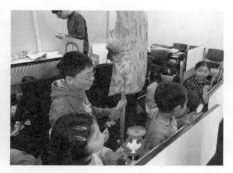

Figure 4. Creating puppets   Figure 5. Rehearsal

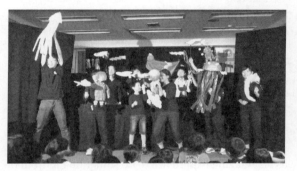

Figure 6. Puppet show performance

4. Evaluating the Puppet Show Program

Here we look at how the Matsui family felt about the puppet show program after it ended after three years of the activity through an interview with Saki. She first provided her honest opinion regarding how the activity the group engaged in differed from what she had imagined.

"I thought it would be more something like they would practice a play that had already been selected, using puppets that had already been made. Then I heard they would make their own puppets, create their own story...basically, if they didn't do it on their own, it wouldn't get done. And I thought that was really amazing. If it weren't like that, we'd still feel like visitors, always just doing what we would be told and then just going home when it would be done. That there is why (the children) are saying they want to keep doing it."

As previously mentioned, the Matsui family felt as they were being treated like "visitors" when they attended a social gathering for evacuees before taking part in the puppet show program. Because the experience necessitated a passive response, participants were hampered from interacting with each other and they didn't feel as if they could settle in. It is likely that other evacuees participating in such social gatherings had similar experiences to some extent. Those holding the social gatherings apparently came to understand this situation and recognized it as an issue that needed to be resolved. According to the 2013 Spring Special Edition of the Fukutama Dayori, the information magazine aimed at disaster victims who had evacuated to Saitama Prefecture, some organizers, for example, noted that the "support/supported" relationship had to be transformed, because it was difficult for evacuee participants to express negative opinions about what was being provided to them when the services were being offered with an excess amount of care. Of the social gatherings we observed, we found some that had dealt with this issue by emphasizing the involvement of participants in the organization of the social gathering, e.g. by having them take over handling of the reception desk and by filling various other roles.

In our puppet show program, participants were invited to produce everything from scratch, from creating a script to creating their own puppets. We saw that this accordingly left a good impression on the Matsui family, which had the experience of being treated like visitors at previous other gatherings. Continuing on, Saki also described what the program meant to the children.

"The children also thought it was an amazing experience to do something in front of other people. That's something that we couldn't give them at home, so having a place like that and an experience like that was really great. And the fact that they were taken on the trips, away from the parents, and not even a school trip…I think the fact that they were able to do that shows how much they've grown."

We see how Saki believes that taking part in the puppet show program and performing plays has helped her children grow as people. That change can apparently also be seen in their everyday lives. For example, after the puppet show program ended, Matsui daughters Hana and Yuki were selected to perform in a recital at their elementary school. It seems that both girls ran actively. They also apparently decided to run for the roles in their class. We were able to see both the surprise and joy in her expression – "because they never did that kind of thing before" – when she told us this during later discussions. Her statements suggest that she too found the puppet play program to be a meaningful experience due to the small changes she witnessed in her children that she interpreted as being due to their having participated in the program. She also mentioned that one thing she found unfortunate was that, once the program finished, the other families stopped coming out to meet them, so the Matsui family was unable to build deeper relationships with the other families through meeting on holidays, etc.

5. Reflecting on Three Years of Activities

It was previously mentioned that the objectives of this program were to (1) help evacuee families build interpersonal networks in their new communities; and (2) to observe and support child development. Finally, here we review the extent to which those objectives were attained. We will also consider the overall meaning of the puppet show program as a form of social gathering aimed at evacuees.

First, in terms of building networks, it is thought that the experience was a beneficial means of support for children living in an unfamiliar area in that they were able to build interpersonal relationships with adults and with children their own age outside of their family and schools. On the other hand, the parents – particularly Saki – felt that relationships couldn't be built through the puppet shows due to the low frequency. Participating families were unable to connect, but the relationships continue both in public and private with the university student staff and individuals from Nouiku Network who helped guide the puppet shows. It is thought that the Matsui family takes some encouragement from the fact that there are people in the community to which they evacuated with whom they spent time together over three years.

Next, in terms of child development, it may not be possible to evaluate the success of this objective at the current point in time. However, as a form of social gathering, it is thought that there was some significance to having the chance to watch over these young and adolescent children over a period of three years. As we shared time with them, we too may have come to have some importance as role models for the children.

As previously discussed, these social gatherings were designed to provide a place for people in similar situations and with similar issues and goals to spend time together, communicating, and therefore they can be seen as a type of self-help group. We have positioned the puppet show program as a type of social gathering as well, and participants included not only evacuees, but other local residents, people connected to the university, and people coming from a variety of other perspectives. That point is where our group differs from the original definition of "self-help group." Regarding the selection of food to serve at the barbecue, differences surfaced regarding the difference in perspective and thinking between evacuees and non-evacuees, forcing us to reconsider how much care must be taken when engaging in such activities. It is possible that some participants may have experienced emotional pain. However, at the very least, when we considered it from the perspective of providing children with a place to interact with others in the communities to which they had evacuated, we did not necessarily think that social gatherings must be for people "in the same situation and sharing similar problems and goals." For example, we believe that we saw some definite growth among the children highlighted here, due to their having taken part in the program, visited various places, and connected with people of various viewpoints, as an opportunity other than school events. We believe that we will learn how significant our social gathering activities were to the children and other family members who took part once those children grow into adults. As of the spring of 2018, the Matsui daughter had already lived for longer in their new communities than they had in Fukushnima. We will maintain this long-term outlook and hope to be able to confirm these points in the future.

IV. Concluding remarks

The evacuation from the nuclear power plant accident took away much from the victims of the disaster, part of which perhaps included their senses of independence and vitality. This is not limited to adult evacuees, but also applies to children. We in the puppet show program supported evacuee families in gaining back their own independence.

The extraordinary circumstances involved with an evacuation place a burden on evacuees in various ways. It may be necessary to specify evacuee needs and issues threatening them in order to think about what sort of support should be offered next. However, considering the issue from a psychological perspective, there may also be value in clarifying factors that can contribute to evacuee mental health. The puppet show program can possibly be used as a model example of an activity that can contribute to the mental well-being of evacuee families, and particularly children, through the opportunity to meet various other people in the community.

References

Gartner, A., Riessman, F., 1977. Self-Help in Human Services. Jossey-Bass Publishers, Hiroaki, K., (Trans.), 1985. *Serufu-Herupu Grūpu no riron to jissai*. [Self-Help Group Theory and Practice.], Kawashima Shoten.

Harada, S., Nishikido, M., 2015. *Kengai hinansha shien no genjyō to kadai: Saitama-ken no jirei kara*. [Current situations and problems with support out-of-prefecture evacuees: Cases from Saitama Prefecture.], In: Kansei Gakuin University Institute of Disaster Area Revitalization, et al., (Ed.), *Genpatsu Hinan Hakusyo*. [Nuclear Accident Evacuation White Paper.], Jimbun Shoin, pp. 17-39.

Hirata, S., Ishijima, K., Mochida, R., Negayama, K., 2013. *Shinsai hinan kazoku no shien kasasagi projekuto no katsudō*. [Support families evacuating earthquakes: activities of the *Kasasagi* Project.], In: Tsujiuchi, T., (Ed.), *Gajyumaru teki shien no susume – Hitori hitori no kokoro ni yorisou*. [Recommendations of Banyan-like Support – Getting closer to each individual.], Waseda University Booklet, After the Disaster 31, Waseda University Press, pp. 17-39.

Ito, T., 2009. *Serufu-herupu grūpu no jiko monogatari ron: arukohorizumu to shibetsu taiken wo rei ni*. [Self-narrative theory of self-help groups: As exemplified by experiences with alcoholism and bereavement.], Harvest.

Matsuzaki, Y., 2008. *Gakkō kyōiku ni okeru ningyō geki no kyōiku teki igi to kadai –Iida-shi no gakkō ni okeru ningyō geki katsudō jyūjitsu no tame ni*. [Educational signifi-cance and issues in puppet shows in school education: Improving puppet the-ater activities at schools in Iida City.], *Iida Women's Junior College Bulletin*, 25, 61-75.

Mochida, R., Shiraishi, Y., Hirata, S., Ishijima, K., Negayama, K., 2012. *Shinsai hinan sha kōryū kai no jittai chōsa: Kodomo wo taishō to shita kōryū kai no arikata wo megutte*. [Field study of disaster evacuee social gatherings: Examining social gatherings aimed at Children.], Collected Research Grant Papers, 48, Meiji Yasuda Mental Health Foundation, pp. 38-46.

Mochida, R., Shiraishi, Y., 2016. *Jisyu hinan kazoku ni taisuru shien no jirei teki kentō: Kodomo wo taisyō to shita kōryū katsudō no kiroku kara*. [From records of social gatherings aimed at children.], In: Ando, K., Matsui, Y., (Ed.), (supervisor), *Shinsai go no oyako wo sasaeru*. [The Supporting parents and Children after the disaster.], Seishin Shobō, pp.49-64.

Noguchi, Y., 2005. *Naratīvu no rinsyō syakai gaku*. [Clinical sociology of narratives.], Keisō Shobō.

Shinsai Shien Network Saitama, 2013. *Hinan no ima to korekara: hinan sha gurūpu rīdā zadan kai*. [The Present and Future of the Evacuation: Roundtable discussion with evacuee group leaders.], *Fukutama Dayori Spring Special Edition*, 6-9.

Tsujiuchi, T., 2012. *Saitama-ken shinsai hinan ankēto chōsa syūkei kekka hōkokusyo*. [Saitama Prefecture Earthquake Evacuation Questionnaire Survey Results Report.], (Third Report Revision), The 10th Saitama Prefecture Earthquake Disaster Council.

84   Part I - 4

Tsujiuchi, T., Masuda, K., 2014. *Saitama Tokyo shinsai hinan ankēto chōsa syūkei kekka hōkokusyo.* [Saitama-Tokyo Earthquake Evacuation Questionnaire Survey Results Report.], (Third Report), *Simposiumu: Syutoken hinan sha no seikatsu saiken e no michi.* [Roadmap to rebuilding the lives of evacuees in the metropolitan Tokyo area.], 58.

*This chapter has translated based on the paper (Mochida and Shiraishi, 2016) in the book "Supporting parents and Children after the disaster " (Ando and Matsui, 2016) published by the Japanese Psychological Association (JPA), and revised it. With regard to the English translation and publication, we have obtained approval of the authors and supervising editor (JPA).

5 Physical Health / Community Health / Environmental Health

The Fukushima Support Project

Development of radiological surveys to support the building of safer environments

Hidetsugu Katsuragawa PhD[*1][*2] *(Nuclear Physics),*
Taisuke Katsuragawa PhD[*3][*4] *(Clinical Psychology)*

Key words: Fukushima support project, nuclear accident, radiation dose rate, radiation contamination levels, hot spot finder

I. Outline of Fukushima Support Project activities

The April 18, 2015 episode of NHK's ETV Special was titled "The Endless Battle – Report on a Fukushima Support Project," and in it, we introduced people to the work we do(1). The program introduced the project members, talked about our activities, position, and attitude, gave a look at volunteer work being done, and described how by the fifth spring since the Fukushima nuclear accident, we were still routinely visiting Fukushima three days a month. The program also explained how the average project member age was 66.6 years old. Perhaps it was just the sense of humor of the producers, but it is rare to repeat people's ages three times over the course of a program. Perhaps they wanted to tell people about our work as relatively older scientists. It has sort of become a regular topic of conversation for the team. Three years have already passed since the program aired, so I supposed our average age must be up to 70 years old.

Our endless battle continues. The survey done between May 9 and 11 2018 was the 51st. We first started working through the project in May 2013, meaning that after a full five years of work, we visited Fukushima an average of roughly ten times a year.

[*1] Professor Emeritus, Toho University
[*2] Visiting Researcher, Waseda Institute of Medical Anthropology on Disaster Reconstruction (WIMA)
[*3] Associate Professor, Faculty of Human Sciences, Waseda University
[*4] Waseda Institute of Medical Anthropology on Disaster Reconstruction (WIMA)

The five central members of the project are Ikuro Anzai (Professor Emeritus, Radiation Protection Studies, Ritsumeikan University); Hidetsugu Katsuragawa (Professor Emeritus, Nuclear Physics, Toho University); Osamu Sato (Professor, Health Education Studies, Fukushima College); Toshihide Yamaguchi (Radiation Measurement Technologies, SWR Co., Ltd.); Toshio Hayakawa (Radiation Measurement Technologies, Taiyo Engineering Joint Venture Company). This is little space to talk about how the group came together, but before the March 11, 2011 nuclear accident, the authors were only acquainted with Anzai. In other words, the group would have never come together had the nuclear accident not occurred. Immediately after the accident, there likely were a number of support groups like ours, but as far as I know, we are the only group that continues to do volunteer work.

Our work has only one goal: to propose and put into practice concrete, feasible means of obtaining a factual understanding of the state of radiation contamination and exposure, helping reduce anxiety among victims, and lowering radiation exposure (i.e. minimizing risk). We are also working to provide a sincere response to people's uncertainty about their everyday lives and other issues. This too is a part of our mission.

II. The Fundamental Stance and Fundamental Perception of the Fukushima Support Project team

A report is put together after each monthly survey is complete, and it is published by the Anzai Science & Peace Office (ASAP). The entire report is compiled by hand by Ikuro Anzai, and it is mainly sent to the individuals and organizations who ordered the radiation surveys be conducted at the locations the project visits. These reports are considered to be private and are not released to the public. Each report contains the following text laying out our Fundamental Stance and Fundamental Perception.

> "We visit the disaster area and go to nursery schools, elementary schools, and other public facilities, residential areas and homes for which a request has been received. There we conduct an environmental survey of radiation levels, then come up with concrete proposals that are as practical as possible on methods of reducing exposure and minimizing risk. We consider the worries of the victims, as we aim to improve their situation."

> "Our fundamental position is that lower radiation exposure is better. We practice four methods to protect people from radiation exposure: 1. Decontamination, 2. Shielding, 3. Increasing distance from the contamination source, and 4. Reducing exposure time. This is how we aim to achieve our goal of minimizing victim exposure as much as possible."

The Fukushima Support Project   87

Our team works with an implicit understanding of these principles. In addition, we also continue to avoid delving too deeply into issues that are a matter of scientific debate. For example, we try to avoid referring to issues such as the health effects of low radiation levels, annual radiation dosage limits, or whether or not nose bleeds were caused by the nuclear accident, an issue made famous by the comic, *Oishinbo*. The Fukushima Support Project was even announced on the previously-mentioned NHK program, ETV Special: "Do not underestimate the situation. Do not be overly afraid. Keep your fear rational." We never force "safety" on residents, while we never overemphasize the "danger." In the end, it is always the residents themselves who must make the decision. As radiation experts, we offer objective information, then respect resident decisions, and work to give them the support they need.

Based on this fundamental stance, upon request, we visit nursery and elementary schools, public facilities, private homes, private lots and farms, where we investigate radiation levels in the environment. We determine the radiation contamination levels and recommend practical methods of reducing exposure. In addition, we also offer consultations and learning activities designed to respond to victim worries. Thus far, we have conducted investigations in the following cities, towns, and villages: Fukushima, Date, Nihonmatsu, Motomiya, Koriyama, Iitate, Minamisoma, Namie, Futaba, Okuma, Tomioka, Naraha, and Iwaki. We have visited 24 nursery schools, kindergartens, and elementary schools, and if we include parks and other public facilities that number passes 30.

III. The first measurements of environmental radiational levels

Our work began with a survey of radiation levels in the area around Sakura Hoikuen, a nursery school in Fukushima City's Watari neighborhood. In more specific terms, we investigated the levels on the student walking course, the use of which had been prohibited since the nuclear accident. We decided to conduct the investigation because we sympathized with the school's passionate teachers, including the head teacher, who told us how the school believes that walking is a necessary part of helping children grow up strong, and that they wanted to reopen the course if they could. For all the surveys, we provide a general summary of the results directly after we finish our measurements, then from the following month, we hold briefings/consultations. Sakura Hoikuen was able to reopen their walking course in October 2013, two and a half years after the nuclear accident. That day, the then-head teacher sent the following email, and included photographs.

"Today, the two-year-olds left the school grounds to go for a walk. It was the first walk they've ever been on. Please take a look at the attached photos. They were a bit nervous when they left, but they were all smiles when they returned. I think we'll all

101 students out for a walk after Sports Day is finished."
We actually visited them that day, and it was a truly moving sight (Sakura Hoikuen, 2014).

Following Sakura Hoikuen, we began to receive requests from new nursery schools to test their walking paths every month. Through word of mouth, we started receiving requests from others as well, including requests to test areas around the homes of people connected to the nursery schools. The work we were doing eventually began to expand into testing areas like school routes for elementary schools, areas around public facilities, and more. The requests came not only from Fukushima City, but from all of the municipalities on the list above, including designated "Difficult-to-Return" zones such as the Tsushima area of Namie, and parts of Okuma, Futaba, and Iitate, and we responded with our radiation level surveys.

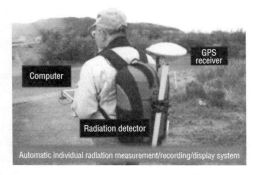

Figure 1. Measuring levels with a hot spot finder

Radiation was measured in terms of air dose rate (μSv/h) using the hot spot finder (HSF) seen in Figure 1 (made by Japan Shield Technical Research Co., Ltd.) An HSF system combines a scintillator using cesium iodide (CsI) crystals, a Global Positioning System (GPS) receiver, and a user computer. A user can simply walk around and color-coded radiation levels for the area will be displayed on a map on the computer's screen.

When measurements are taken at a private home and a "hot spot" (an area with a high radiation dose rate) is found, radioactive contamination of the soil in the area is measured (in Bq/kg). In the case of a farm, the soil in the rice paddies and fields is tested, as is radioactivity concentration in water, farm produce, etc. The reason we were able to respond immediately to the May 2013 request from Nursery School Sakura Hoikuen with this automatic radiation measurement/recording/display system is due to the development work conducted by project members like Yamaguchi and Hayakawa. We started using this system in April 2013 and managed to test radiation levels over more than 200 km of walking distance in Fukushima City. This was an enormous achievement. It is possible that no other survey in the city has covered such a long distance with such precision. Moreover, we measured the air dose rates three years running from 2013 to 2015, during the same March-April time frame, covering essentially the same route each time. The results can be found plotted on the map in Figure 2. It wouldn't be unfair to call this use of the cutting-edge HSF system, alongside the sheer physical strength and perseverance required to conduct the surveys, an unparalleled achievement. Great scientific value could also be found in gaining an understanding of the state of contamination within Fukushima City, and of the effectiveness and testing of decontamination efforts. The work of the Fukushima Support Project is not being done with research in mind, so at this stage, our accumulated data is only being used in reports, for personal communications with those requesting surveys, and for learning sessions. However, we are convinced that we have accumulated enough data that it could even withstand the rigor of scientific verification.

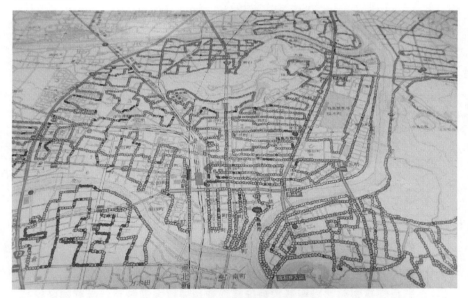

Figure 2. Example of radiation dose measurements results in Fukushima City (acquired in March 2013)

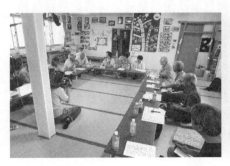

Figure 3. Briefing session on June 19, 2016 with individuals living in Onodai Residences in Soma after evacuating from Iitate. Meeting covered by NHK.

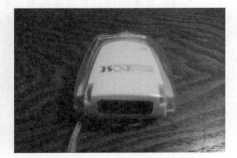

Figure 4. MiniDose (manufactured by U.S. company RAE Systems, Inc.)

IV. Measuring radiation in areas with high air dose rates and measuring individual external exposure levels

When conducting radiation measurements around homes in both urban and farming areas, we often received requests to measure radiation levels within the home, likely due to concerns regarding how much radiation the individuals were being exposed to every day. Briefing sessions are held alongside consultations and lectures (Fig. 3) to report on results obtained during the surveys conducted one or two months previously. At those sessions, a common concern people have was about how much radiation they had been exposed to. The Fukushima Support Project generally advised worried individuals to wear a personal dosage meter for a month to obtain data, and we lent out MiniDose dosimeters (Fig.4) to those who wished to wear them. Mini-Dose dosimeters are small (55mm by 65 mm in size) and they are an important tool in the Fukushima Support Project team's toolbox. It is an excellent device that detects the presence of radiation using CsI crystals and measures exposure rates on a daily, weekly, monthly, or annual basis. Normally, they are used as day monitors, and we ask borrowers to record their activities.

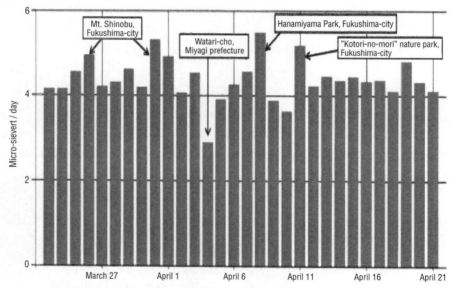

Figure 5. Example of data gathered using MiniDose (Subject K, a resident of Fukushima City's Koganeyama neighborhood)

The graph in Figure 5 shows an example of data gathered by one individual using a MiniDose (Subject K, a resident of Fukushima City's Koganeyama neighborhood). The data shows exposure rates for a period from March 23 to April 21, 2016. Daily exposure was approximately 4.4 µSv. Comparing the data to Subject K's activity logs, we find that Subject K went for hikes on Mt. Shinobu, in Kotori-no-mori, and Mt. Jumanko, all of which are said to have high air dosage levels. On those days, the dosimeter measured higher levels of exposure, thereby reflecting the air dosage rates in those areas. In contrast, we find a lower rate on the day Subject K went outside the prefecture. This information suggests that the MiniDose dosimeter provides accurate measurements of changing radiation exposure levels.

One of the authors always wears a MiniDose dosimeter while conducting radiation surveys in Fukushima, but he also wears it in regular life as well in order to record everyday radiation exposure levels. The MiniDose dosimeter does not have many functions, but it does contain a calendar function, which allows for the daily collection of exposure level values as shown in Figure 5. At midnight, the display is set to zero, after which the 24-hour accumulated dose is recorded. This data can then be transferred to a PC to create a graph like Figure 5.

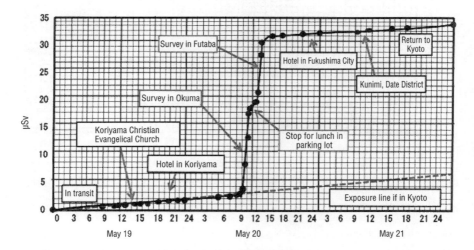

Figure 6. Accumulated radiation dose during May 2016 survey

In addition, when asked to conduct surveys in Difficult-to-Return zones and other areas, by setting confirmation times and making notes of exposure rates up to those times, we are able to create accumulated exposure charts like that shown in Figure 6. During surveys, we set time intervals for when MiniDose values should be read in accordance with the air dose rates for the area being surveyed, then record the time confirmed and accumulated exposure in our notes. These records are placed in chart form with time on the horizontal axis and total accumulated exposure on the vertical axis, which results in a graph like Figure 6 (excerpted from the May 2016 report).

Looking at this graph, we find that there was a total exposure of approximately 33 µSv during the survey period (three days), and that the vast majority of that exposure was accumulated while measuring radiation levels in Okuma and Futaba, both of which are designated Difficult-to-Return zones. This data corresponds to the exposure accumulated during that period, but it makes sense to assume that other members of the project are experiencing similar levels of exposure. Near the center of the graph we see a sudden spike between the times of 9:00 and 15:00 on May 20, but in the middle of that spike we see that the slope of the line is reduced somewhat at the point that we stopped in the parking lot at a highway interchange to have lunch in the car. Such details make the graph even more interesting.

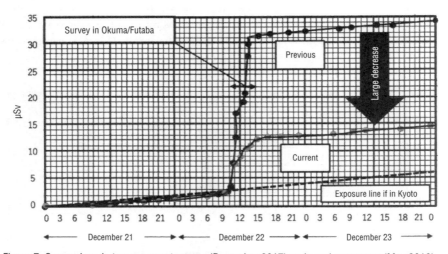

Figure 7. Comparison between current survey (December 2017) and previous survey (May 2016)

Figure 7 shows a comparison of exposure data gathered in December 2017 (the current survey) to data gathered a year and a half previously in May 2016 (the previous survey). The routes followed for each survey were essentially the same. Exposure dropped to around 40% of the previous level. This is thought to be a clear result of the decay of cesium 134.

Figure 8 illustrates how exposure doses were accumulated during the December 2017 survey in the form of a graph showing radiation dose rate change over time. The analysis was performed by Michito Kawata, who joined the team in June 2016. It shows a sharp peak at the time the dosimeter entered the Okuma/Futaba area on December 22 between 10 and 11 AM.

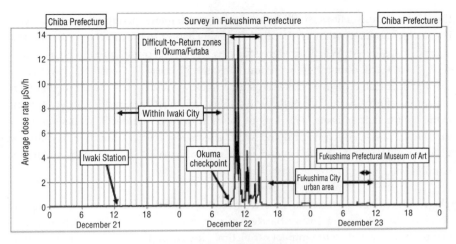

Figure 8. Radiation dose rate change during December 2017 survey

V. Conclusion

This concludes our summary of the more than 50 surveys conducted over five years by the Fukushima Support Project. The five members of the project team were aided by a diverse range of individuals who lent their support when needed, including: Yoshiharu Hashizume (freelance engineer/radiation measurement technologies); Michito Kawata (freelance engineer/data analysis techniques); Yuriko Shimano (ASAP offices); Hiroyuki Yoshino (Shalom Disaster Relief Center Fukushima); Masao Takagaki (neurosurgeon, cultural anthropology); Yasunori Koyabu (retired high school teacher/physics and astronomy); and many, many more.

This report was unable to cover how the five-member project team came to be founded, or the activities of many of our supporters. In addition, we were unable to discuss the many opinions we received from victims during consultations, briefings, and learning sessions, or the comments we received on site during surveys and in other forums. Finally, we were unable to describe how radioactive concentrations were measured in soil, in vegetables, fruit, and other farm products, or in leaves, grass, or local water supplies. This leaves us with the opportunity to cover these details in the future.

The on-site surveys were conducted more than 50 times, almost monthly, and during them we investigated how much radiation victims were really exposed to, and to what extent the areas in which they live have been contaminated by radioactive matter. Our aim was to provide concrete proposals on methods that will further reduce radiation exposure. However, the authors were particularly struck by something they learned during the surveys from speaking with many victims about the effect of the nuclear accident: namely, that there is a new aspect to the effect of radiation that must be considered. When we were studying the effects of radiation in an academic setting, we learned that there were four effects:1. Physical, 2. Genetic, 3. Psychological, and 4. Social. However, this Fukushima nuclear accident has taught us that there is another effect – 5. the loss of the will to live – an effect shown by victims suffering from such a serious issue. This loss of the will to live, number 5, seems similar to numbers 3 and 4, psychological and social effects respectively, but there is one clear difference. These effects are beyond what we as a survey support team are able to handle.

The results of our research up to now have shown us that the effects of the nuclear accident do not simply end at the "effect of radiation." We strongly feel that they extend beyond that to the impact on victim's life overall, and to the community in general. The Fukushima Support Project was launched with the goal of providing support to the overall development of children as people, by reducing the risk of exposure to radioactive substances that continue to plague the areas where people live as much as possible. However, I think it can be said that our perspective was too narrow; perhaps it was beyond our ability to comprehend. On June 14, 2018, the president of TEPCO informed the governor of Fukushima Prefecture that they would like to undertake a concrete review into how to decommission of the reactors at Fukushima Daini Nuclear Power Plant. It is the dream of all the victims we met during this project to build a safe and secure environment for the future. In order to solve the fundamental issues at hand, it is necessary to continue to demand that the planned decommissioning of the reactors is conducted safely and promptly, and to that end, we as a nation must have a broader, more encompassing perspective that allows us to see how the nuclear power issue can be brought to an end. The authors have also had the opportunity to hold half-day study sessions with nuclear reactor experts and doctors specializing in thyroid cancer during our three-day survey trips.

We would like to end this report with some information on the survey conducted in May 2018. This survey was conducted at a farm growing perilla in Namie, a designated Difficult-to-Return zone. Subject I from Namie has resumed perilla cultivation, and has a strong desire to produce perilla oil, chili oil, perilla jam, and other products. We conducted environmental surveys of radiation levels and supported soil improvement effects from June 2018, when seeds were planted, until the harvest in late October. The endless battle of radiation scientists to help build a safer environment will continue.

References

Katsuragawa, H., 2016. *Fukushima Projekuto chōsa ni yoru gaibu hibaku senryō no sokutei.* [Measurement of external exposure levels by Fukushima Project surveys.], Nuclear and Energy-Related Information Center, *NERIC News*, 382, 4 – 5.

NHK: ETV Special, 2015. *Owari naki tatakai – Aru Fukushima shien purojekuto no kiroku.* [The Endless Battle –Report on a Fukushima Support Project.], aired April 18, Available from: 2015 http://www.nhk.or.jp/etv21c/file/2015/0418.html.

Sakura Hoikuen (Ed.), Anzai, I., Omiya, I., 2014. *Sore demo Sakura wa Saku: Fukushima – Watari anohi kara Hoiku wo tsukuru.* [Still the Cherry Blossoms Bloom: Nurturing children in Watari, Fukushima since that fateful day.], Kamogawa Publishing.

6 Community Health / Cultural Health / Human Security

Citizens Work Together to Overcome Disaster

Yuichi Sekiya PhD[*1][*2] *(Cultural Anthropology, Studies of Development)*

Key words: Fukushima, Chernobyl, collaborative commons, evacuee,
**   interview**

I. "A Paradise Built in Hell" After the Disaster

1. In Fukushima

After the triple disaster of earthquake, tsunami, and nuclear accident rocked Japan on March 11, 2011, as many as 450,000 people were forced to live as evacuees across the country at its peak. Their lives had been shattered, evacuation instructions from the government were incomplete at best, and they suffered from a continuous and overwhelming shortage of information. Residents of the areas surrounding Tokyo Electric Company's Fukushima Daiichi Nuclear Power Plant even evacuated to areas with greater dispersion of radioactive materials due to the effects of the prevailing winds at the time of the incident. What sorts of information were evacuees using to base their decisions on in such an urgent situation? What opportunities did they have? How did they evacuate? The author and fellow researchers conducted an interview-based survey in the city of Tsukuba and discovered that evacuees had moved as many as three to five times in the year before settling down in Tsukuba, and some subjects had moved as many as eight times[1]. Government instructions and evacuation measures were of no use in the evacuation, and many relied on the family, friends, and strangers they met while evacuating.

---

*1 Associate Professor, Graduate Program on Human Security, Graduate School of Arts and Sciences, The University of Tokyo
*2 Visiting Researcher, Waseda Institute of Medical Anthropology on Disaster Reconstruction (WIMA)

---

1) The interview data referenced in this chapter was based upon the interview survey conducted in Tsukuba. A total of 49 of the 50 records obtained were analyzed using NVivo qualitative data analysis software (Ver.11).

98   Part I - 6

People able to rely on their own personal networks were, the longer they lived as evacuees, more likely to feel an emotional drive to avoid being a further burden on others. Fukushima residents who evacuated to Tsukuba had fled under varying circumstances, but it is known that to reach Tsukuba, many evacuees worked together to provide mutual aid, or depended on relatives, friends, and others connected to them to obtain information. Moreover, the data also indicated that many evacuees felt the need to avoid being a burden on others while evacuated, and as much as possible, made the effort to resolve their problems on their own or by obtaining official support. In this way, citizens began working together to overcome the issues caused by the disaster in an organic and voluntary way immediately after the disaster struck.

2. In Marseille

At the time of the Tohoku earthquake, I was in Marseille, France. Since April 2010, I had been working as a visiting researcher at the anthropology laboratory in the School of Medicine at the University of the Mediterranean in the city, and the plan was to be there for a year in total. There is an eight-hour time difference between France and Japan, so when the tsunami was generated at 2:46 PM, it was still 6:46 AM in France. However, around 9 AM that day, I left for the laboratory and arrived to find the television on in the office and all the laboratory staff watching the news of the tsunami that had occurred in distant Japan. "Your country is facing a hard time," they told me. However, with the small screen and the announcers speaking in rapid-fire French, I thought it was just one of those rare occasions when a large tsunami had caused some damage at first. After some strong persuasion, I finally came to realize that it wasn't just a minor event.

That Sunday evening, I was on my daily walk and I visited Notre-Dame de la Garde Basilica. When I sat down in a pew, the priest stood before the mic stand beside the altar in the back and began to pray. When the sermon was over, he suddenly said, "Let us now pray for the people of Japan, which has been devastated by an earthquake and tsunami." I was surprised to see such a great number of the citizens of Marseille praying for Japan, and it moved me to tears that took some time to stop. As a developed nuclear power, the people of France had a comparatively good understanding of the seriousness of the Fukushima nuclear power plant accident, and I soon learned that immediately after the earthquake, a large number of rescue teams departed from Marseille airport with humanitarian supplies and equipment to help deal with the nuclear power accident.

In the Fukushima evacuees immediately after March 11, and in the sympathy and desire to assist directed towards Japan I encountered in Marseille, I saw similarities to Rebecca Solnit's "paradise built in hell" i.e. the concept of a disaster utopia. Solnit pointed out that people who experience a large-scale disaster first-hand do not act selfishly in the disaster zone; they do not panic, and do not regress into savagery. In fact, people tend to act altruistically and with compassion (Solnit, 2010) in such tense situations. That phenomenon was witnessed among the Fukushima evacuees discussed earlier in this section. However, my experiences in Marseille showed that this "disaster utopia" is a global phenomenon, in which nameless people are able to turn their thoughts to a difficult situation faced by people in far-flung lands, people with a different language and culture, and with goodwill and a desire to collaborate, are able to act instantly and altruistically to aid them.

II. Citizens working together to overcome disaster

The idea discussed in this article of a coalition of citizens working to overcome disaster in a collaborative society is directly connected to Solnit's "disaster utopia" conditions mentioned above, in which altruistic behavior is promoted, and people work effectively and systematically towards disaster relief and reconstruction. It is a manifestation of humanity's organizational behavior. Here it can be defined as the foundation for goal-oriented, organized behavior and practices in the conditions I encountered while conducting research surveys and educational practice since the disaster.

Social theorist Jeremy Rifkin published a book titled, *The Zero Marginal Cost Society: The internet of things, the collaborative commons, and the eclipse of capitalism* in 2014 (Rifkin, 2014 [2015]). In it, Rifkin said that we in the 21st century are witnessing the collapse of capitalist society and the birth of a shared economy developed within the collaborative commons. The collaborative commons serve to underpin the shared economy. The theories about the rise of the collaborative commons are worthy of our attention. Rifkin believes that the driving force behind that rise is the Internet of Things (IoT), but what is important is that the motivation to realize the collaborative commons and build a shared economy is made possible through IoT, and has spread throughout modern society through a historic series of events. It is the qualitive transformation of humanity and society that is underpinning the effectiveness of technology, which provides only the opportunity to amplify that transformation (Toyama, 2014).

Incidentally, for me, Fukushima Prefecture served as the stage for the formation of a collaborative commons, though before the nuclear accident, it was a relatively unfamiliar place to me – one I visited twice a year for work. After March 11, 2011, I visited Fukushima through my relationship with Toru Shima and Yoshiko Igarashi of Gensousha, a cultural and academic publisher located in Tokyo's Jimbocho neighborhood. From the end of March 2012, I visited the town of Iino multiple times and had the opportunity to speak with volunteers from the town's Social Welfare Council (Sekiya, 2012).

During my trips, I was able to meet and speak with people from Iino; with Sachiko Sato, representative of an NPO called the Fukushima Network for Saving Children from Radiation; Mari Kobayashi, a farmer from the village of Iitate and employee with the local social welfare organization; Nobuyuki Abe, public relations director with the NPO Citizens Radioactivity Monitoring Station; and the previously mentioned Toru Shima from Gensousha. Later on, towards the end of our discussions, I also had the chance to speak with each of them about giving open university seminars as lecturers.

In addition, I obtained information from the people I met during my initial surveys, and on my way home, I went to the Agri Coffee café[2], where I met up with Shuko and Miyuki Ichisawa, from whom I managed to obtain a promise to meet me during my study trip discussed below. This is how the collaborative commons was formed. This chapter will show how collaborative commons functions and will show the successes achieved by citizens working together to overcome disasters through a stage-by-stage description of the discussion I engaged in: university seminars, study trips, evacuee interviews, the Ukraine survey and talks with Shinonome-no-kai.

III. Seminar collaborations

Beginning in April 2011, staff members in the University of Tokyo's Human Security Program began offering HSP seminars, a series of public seminars aimed at discussing the Tohoku earthquake and the nuclear power plant accident in Fukushima. Details on the seminars offered by the aforementioned individuals can be found in chronological order below.

> HSP Seminars: Earthquakes, Nuclear Power and Human Security.
> May 24, 2012
> 11th Seminar: Protecting the children of Fukushima from radiation
> Sachiko Sato (Representative, Fukushima Network for Saving Children from Radiation)
>
> November 16, 2012
> 16th Seminar: Fukushima, Iitate – The world is still a beautiful place
> Mari Kobayashi (Iitate farmer & social welfare organization staff)
>
> November 22, 2012

---

2) Details on the origin of Agri Coffee and the history of the Ichisawas in Iitate can be found in the book written by the couple (Ichisawa 2013).

17th Seminar: Fukushima and Human Security
Toru Shima (Representative, Gensousha)

December 2, 2012
18th Seminar: Fukushima Today and What Everyone Should Know
Nobuyuki Abe (Public Relations Director, Citizens Radioactivity Monitoring Station NPO, Fukushima)

What the four individuals who gave the HSP seminars described above shared with the people of Fukushima is that all of them are ordinary citizens, without particular social role. They took action of their own volition, and building ties with other, they all continued to work hard to provide the information and support required by other people facing the same nuclear disaster they were facing. Participant response at each seminar was moderate. What made such high-quality learning experiences possible was that individual citizens came together in a collaborative commons designed to rebuild after the disaster, and create a forum and foundation for excellent study, research and education.

IV. The Fukushima Study Trip

On July 28 and 29, 2012, I travelled to Fukushima with nine undergraduate and graduate student volunteers. The information network had grown since my first visit, and preparations for the study tour, which was meant to coincide with the holding of the Soma Nomaoi events, were supported and made possible by the individuals I met through my own expanded information network (Sekiya, 2012). We conducted another study tour to coincide with the Soma Nomaoi the following year in 2013, and from 2014, I was able to obtain funding support through Grants-in-Aid, which allowed us to focus on research surveys during the Fukushima study trips. The list below provides a summary of the study trips conducted from 2014 onwards.

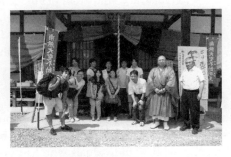

Figure 1. Fukushima Study Trip

November 22-23, 2014 (Four researchers, three students)
Field trip to areas of Minamisoma damaged by the tsunami, attended picture story play by Mihoko Murakami of the town of Shinchi

October 31-November 1, 2015 (Six researchers, five students)

Visit to offices of Tomioka Association for the Discussion of March 11, study tour of the town of Naraha (visited residence of Tsukuba evacuee Takeo Igari)

March 5-6, 2016 (Five researchers, seven students)
Attended lecture of Fukushima Studies at Sakura no Seibo Junior College, visited Agri Coffee café and village of Ten-ei

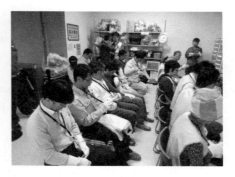

Figure 2. Inside the power plant

September 5-6, 2016 (Ten researchers/volunteers, three students)
Tours of Kajima Corporation JV offices, Iwaki City Hall, and grounds of TEPCO Fukushima Daiichi Nuclear Power Plant

November 3-5, 2017 (Fourteen researchers/volunteers)
Visits to Decontamination Information Plaza, Agri Coffee, Minamisoma, and Tomioka, and study tour of Fukushima 30-year Project

The Fukushima residents I worked with during the study trips formed the collaborative commons for learning that ensured the trips would be fruitful and fulfilling.

V. Evacuee collaborations

The research surveys that formed the foundation of my study of the victims of the Fukushima nuclear power plant disaster began in January 2013 and continued for ten months with 50 individuals who had evacuated to Tsukuba City. Interviews were conducted by Naoki Takeda, the author's collaborative researcher, and by Tsukuba Gakuin University, myself, and the other members of the University of Tokyo HSP team. At that time, Takeda was working as a head of local NPO who was functioning as safety net creator for the evacuees. At the same time, Takeda was teaching life planning at Tsukuba Gakuin University. I was in a University of Tokyo graduate course and looking for access to evacuees, while Takeda was looking for an opportunity to hear evacuee opinions in order to build a safety net for such individuals. Keiko Iwasaki was then a graduate student at the University of Tokyo, and she was asked to serve as the primary researcher on behalf of the university. Iwasaki was able to complete her master's degree thesis based upon surveys conducted on 22 households (Iwasaki, 2013), then began her doctoral studies. Her 2017 doctoral dissertation provided a valuable look at her development of more quantitative analysis methods and consideration of issues concerning mental health care (Iwasaki, 2017).

Returning momentarily to 2013, including the 22 interviews conducted by Iwasaki, a total of 50 interviews were conducted up to the end of October that year. The data gathered covered the evacuation route individuals followed from immediately after the disaster until settling in Tsukuba, narratives about their experiences, and feelings they had and issues they had faced since moving to Tsukuba. Much was learned from these interviews. Evacuee testimonies taught us that the national and local government system they would have relied on and which they would have expected to protect them in normal times had collapsed around them. They were separated from the people and places they knew, and knew little about what was happening. In that situation, these individuals frantically made use of their own personal connections (e.g. relatives, friends, acquaintances, and people they met in Tsukuba) to finally find peace in Tsukuba. This shows us that even when people are anxious and facing various problems, they will still search work, schools, and ways to connect with neighbors in order to establish a new home. This is why something like Takeda's safety net is so necessary. Moreover, the interviews transcended the original research objective in that they provided a means for evacuees and Takeda to connect, and thereby led to the future building of a safety net in Tsukuba.

VI. Ukrainian collaborations

Naoki Takeda and I travelled to Ukraine from September 5-12, 2014, and visited the Chernobyl Nuclear Power Plant and people connected to it. Below is a list of the main organizations and individuals interviewed during that trip.

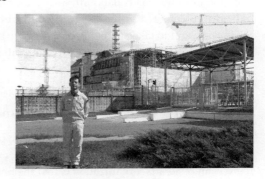

Figure 3. Research in Chernobyl

-Zemlyaki (people from the same area) – Disabled citizens organization of Chernobyl
-Chernobyl victims fund
-5-2 Citizens group for acute radiation diseases
-Zhytomyr police and fire victims group
-Chernobyl Hostage charity fund
-Chernobyl victims fund
-Painting class for children in Zhytomyr
-National University of Agriculture in Zhytomyr, Professor Микола Дідух
-Employee of Ukrainian television network STB – Natalia Yeskova Pogorielova

104   Part I - 6

Takeda wanted to visit Chernobyl in order to build the Tsukuba City safety net for nuclear evacuees from Fukushima Prefecture. His aim was to learn from the victims of the Chernobyl nuclear accident, and harness what he learned to build his network for evacuees in Tsukuba (Takeda, 2015). For around a week in September 2014, we rushed between Kiev, Zhytomyr, and Chernobyl, and we were able to gather only fragments of information, but with the help of the ethnography written by Adriana Petryna, we were able to gain a better understanding of how people connected to the accident struggled through those turbulent times. She states that in the post-Chernobyl disaster area there emerged a concept she called biological citizenship, a social practice by which Ukrainians demanded rights through their status as victims of the disaster (Petryna, 2016). Sociologist Junji Kayukawa promptly realized the importance of Petryna's research from the perspective of the Japanese people and pointed to the emergence of biological citizens in Fukushima. On that, he said that on one hand, as was emphasized by the media and shown in Ukraine, some victims of the nuclear disaster showed a passive attitude regarding the subject of compensation. However, on the other hand, he emphasized that there were also people who did the opposite, e.g. cool-headed farmers actively measured the extent of contamination due to radioactive substances in their produce and disclosed this information on their own initiative (Kayukawa, 2016).

This chapter discusses the people of Fukushima I met in Fukushima and Tsukuba, and who have formed collaborative commons. They work together to consider how best to implement disaster reconstruction through the interviews, seminars, and study trips, and to take action. As described by Kayukawa, they were able to collaborate with others when necessary by making rational decisions in order to secure their rights as active agents, or biological citizens.

VII. Working with the Shinonome-no-kai

After the Chernobyl survey in 2014, I met with people living as evacuees a little close to home. I visited the Shinonome residence for public servants in Kotō-ku, where there is an residents' organization called the Shinonome-no-kai that holds "salons", every Tuesday and Thursday from 13:00–15:00. At these salons, evacuees living in the residence can come together and enjoy tea and snacks while sharing information or engage in some simple creative activities such as handicrafts, and outsiders are free to join in. Support is provided by the Kotō-ku Social Welfare Council, and it is run by resident volunteers. I took the day off of my duties at the university to visit the salon one Tuesday in October 2014. However, while I was able to speak with people, I was unable to interview anyone. In contrast to the Tsukuba City interviews I conducted with Naoki Takeda, it was difficult to build a work-based give-and-take relationship with the people of the Shinonome-no-kai.

Citizens Work Together to Overcome Disaster 105

In 2015, I became advisor for a student named Xue Yang, and she essentially couldn't speak Japanese. She had studied anthropology at a Chinese university and experienced the 2008 Sichuan earthquake, so she wanted to use her experiences to interview victims of the Fukushima nuclear power plant disaster and write a research paper on her findings. Yang was driven to make the most of her limited time at the university, only two years, so recruited university friends, employed part-time interpreters, and began conducting long interviews with the elderly people of the Shinonome-no-kai. She was saved by the organization's then-vice-chairman, Yuji Takahashi. Takahashi served as the contact point for visitors wanting to take part in the Shinonome-no-kai. Yang would set up interviews, and when difficulties arose, Takahashi would lend a hand.' There were surely members of the Shinonome-no-kai who felt as if they were being forced to take part and who tired of the interviews. However, Yang's master's thesis, titled *The Locked Doors: An Anthropological Study of Fukushima Evacuees in Tokyo*, showed that the more than 1,000 evacuees living at the residence were unused to life in the apartment-like setting and spent their days quietly behind "locked doors." Her work illuminated how such individuals to become accustomed to life in the city through strengthening the bonds with others from their hometowns during salons and other events, and through periodically leaving the residence to engage with people from Tokyo. "Bonds" and "adaptation" became the keywords of her thesis, and she was able to clearly illustrate the inner conflict that resulted in evacuees in Tokyo living in a state of limbo, unable to escape (Yang, 2016). Yang worked hard on her thesis, but the support of the Shinonome-no-kai was an important part of her success.

VIII. Summary

Since March 11, 2011, the evacuees of Fukushima have built a collaborative network they could rely on during the evacuation process made up of other individuals trapped in the same situation they were in. The technological and environmental catalysts of this global era have given it the potential to spread from the temporary, limited form such as that exemplified by Solnit's "disaster utopia", and be reborn as a more sustainable and ubiquitous collaborative commons.

We also see that collaborative commons in the form of citizens willing to work together to overcome disaster, both in the compassionate desire to help I witnessed in Marseille, and in the connections that emerged to serve as a foundation for more concrete learning, through the research and educational activities aimed at helping rebuild from the disaster – including the University of Tokyo seminars, study trips, and interview surveys – which were made possible through the expansion of my network by conducting surveys in Fukushima Prefecture. These forms of collaboration were seen among the citizens of Ukraine after the Chernobyl nuclear power plant accident, and in Fukushima, Japan since March 11, 2011.

The Fukushima evacuees formed new bonds in their new homes in Tsukuba, and the former Fukushima residents of the Shinonome-no-kai became accustomed to life in Tokyo. We see in that the challenge that must be undertaken to overcome such an unprecedented disaster – the challenge inherent to independently and calmly developing the connections needed to survive in a dispersed, collaborative, and horizontal way.

References

Ichisawa, S., Ichisawa, M., 2013. *Yama no Kōhīya Iitate 'Aguri' no kiroku*. [Records of the moutain café in Iitate, Agri.], Gensōsha.

Iwasaki, K., 2013. Social Capital and Mental Health among Displaced Residents Due to the Fukushima Nuclear Accident: A Quantitative Assessment of Survey Data from Futaba Town, Fukushima. Master's thesis submitted to the University of Tokyo.

Iwasaki, K., 2017. Social Capital and Mental Health among Displaced Residents from Fukushima. Doctoral Dissertation submitted to the University of Tokyo.

Kayukawa, J., 2016. *Kaisetsu Chernobyl to Fukushima no seibutsu teki shimin ken*. [Commentary on biological citizenship in Chernobyl and Fukushima.], In: Petryna, A., Life Exposed: Biological citizens after Chernobyl. Kayukawa, J., (Sup.Ed.), Morimoto, M., Wakamatsu, F., (Trans.), Jimbun Shoin, pp315-27.

Petryna, A., 2016. *Sarasareta sei: Chernobyl go no seibutsu gaku teki shimin*. [Life Exposed: Biological citizens after Chernobyl.], Kayukawa, J., (Sup.Ed.), Morimoto, M., Wakamatsu, F., (Trans.), Jimbun Shoin.

Rifkin, J., 2014 [2015]. *Genkai hiyō zero syakai: Mono no intānetto to kyōyū gata Keizai no daitō*. [The Zero Marginal Cost Society: The internet of things, the collaborative commons, and the eclipse of capitalism.], NHK Publishing, Inc.

Sekiya, Y., 2012. *Fukushima-ken e no izanai: Manabi no tabi kara no kyōkun*. [Invitation to Fukushima Prefecture – Lessons learned from study trips.], In: *Sōgō Kankyō Gakkai*. [General Tourism Society.] (Ed.), *Fukkō Tsūrizumu*. [Reconstruction Tourism.], Dō Bun kan Shuppan, pp68-75.

Solnit, R., 2010. *Saigai yūtopia: Naze sono toki tokubetsu na kyōdōtai ga tachi agaru noka*. [A Paradise Built in Hell: The Extraordinary Communities that Arise in Disaster.], Takatsuki, S., (Trans.), Aki Shobō.

Toyama, K., 2016. *Tekunorojī wa hinkon wo sukuwanai*. [Can Technology End Poverty?], Yutaka, M., (Trans.), Misuzu Shobō.

Wikipedia, 2012. *Sōma no umaoi*. [The Horse Driver in Soma.], Available from: https://ja.wikipedia.org/wiki/相馬野馬追 [Accessed 16 March 2018]

Yang, X., 2016. The Locked Doors: An Anthropological Study of Fukushima Evacuees in Tokyo. Master's thesis submitted to the University of Tokyo.

Part II

RESEARCH PROJECT

1 Physical Health / Mental Health / Social Health

Mental Health Impact of the Great East Japan Earthquake

Eugene F. Augusterfer LCSW[1] (Telemedicine, Global Mental Health),
Takuya Tsujiuchi MD, PhD[2,3] (Medical Anthropology)

Key words: Great East Japan Earthquake, mental health, PTSD,
psychiatric problem, number of global disasters

I. Introduction

This paper is a follow-up to the paper *High Prevalence of Post-Traumatic Stress Symptoms in Relation to Social Factors in Affected Population One Year after the Fukushima Nuclear Disaster*, published March 2016, PLoS One (Tsujiuchi, T., et al., 2016). Specifically, this paper will examine published papers regarding the lessons learned in the area of mental health impact of the Great East Japan Earthquake. The Great East Japan Earthquake of 2011, GEJE, (9.1 magnitude) represents a combination of a natural disaster and technological disaster. The undersea earthquake triggered a tsunami, which in turn caused a technological disaster (the meltdown of nuclear reactors).

This major disaster caused the death of 15,894 people with over 3,200 people missing, numerous people injured, and more than 321,000 people forced to evacuate their homes. As of February 2017, Japan's Reconstruction Agency reports that about 50,000 evacuees were still living in temporary housing (Live Science, 2017).

The United Nations (2018) reports that disasters, natural and man-made, have caused 68.5 million forcibly displaced persons, 40.3 million internally displaced persons, 25.4 million refugees, and 10 million stateless persons worldwide. The World Bank (2016) reports that in the presence of conflict situations, the psychiatric literature estimates an increase in disorder prevalence explained by high levels of stress that can prompt psychosocial or psychiatric disorders that were previously nonexistent or

---

[1] Director of Telemedicine, Harvard Program in Refugee Trauma (HPRT)
[2] Professor, Faculty of Human Sciences, Waseda University
[3] Director, Waseda Institute of Medical Anthropology on Disaster Reconstruction (WIMA)

dormant. Disasters, both natural and man-made, are on the rise world-wide, as documented by the Centre for Research on the Epidemiology of Disasters, CRED (2016). See figure 1, below.

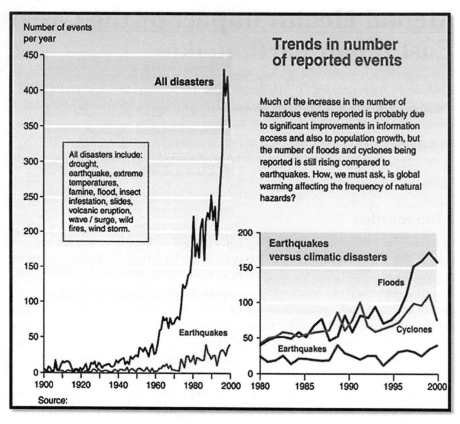

Figure 1. Source: CRED Annual Disaster Statistical Review 2006, 2007.

The need for health and mental health services to address the problems caused by disasters and displacement is well documented. Unipolar depression is number three on the World Health Organization Burden of Disease "Disability Adjusted Life Years (DALYs)" list of global disorders and is number one for women world-wide in the age group of 15 to 44 years. Further, based on current trends, unipolar depression is predicted to be the number one on the burden of disease list world-wide by 2030 (WHO, 2018).

II. Mental Health Impact of Disasters

Disasters, both natural and man-made, affect millions of people around the world every year. Mollica et al. report that mental health is becoming a central issue for public health complex emergencies (Mollica, R.F., et al., 2004). Although temporary symptoms tend to be common in the acute phase of disaster recovery, psychological sequelae can persist for a number of years after a disaster.

Neria and colleagues performed a systematic review of 284 peer-reviewed published studies of the mental health impact of natural disasters and concluded that "PTSD among persons exposed to disasters is substantial" (Neria, Y., et al., 2008). Dai, et al., (2016), preformed a meta-analysis of forty six published articles which examined PTSD rates in 76,101 survivors of earthquakes who met the inclusion criteria. Using a random effects model, the combined incidence of PTSD after earthquakes was 23.66% (Dai, W., et al., 2016).

We will now examine the mental health impact of the GEJE. As reported in our previously published paper, of the 350 households surveyed comprising 187 females and 163 males, the prevalence of PTSD symptoms was extremely high with a mean score of 36.15 as measured with the Impact of Event Scale-Revised (IES-R) Japanese version (Tsujiuchi, T., et al., 2016).

In a study of female college students, a cross-sectional survey was conducted of 310 female students at a college in Fukushima Prefecture, who lived in Fukushima at the time of the GEJE. The study utilized the World Health Organization-Five Well-Being Index and the results indicate that 46.5% of participants reported depressive symptoms (Ito, S., et al., 2018).

In another study of mental health recovery of evacuees and residents from the Fukushima disaster, Orui, M., et al. (2018a) examined factors associated with mental health recovery. The study concluded that there is a positive association between mental health recovery and a desirable lifestyle and social network, particularly with social roles. Specifically, they report that social interaction with friends from pre-disaster periods and social roles defined through daily activities were significantly associated with mental health recovery. However, disaster-related loss of employment and economic hardship were still associated with non-recovered mental health status even when the positive effects of good general subjective health status, regular physical activity, social interaction with friends from pre-disaster periods, and social roles through daily activities on their mental health were considered (Orui, M., et al., 2018b). In an interesting case study, Hori, A., et al. (2018) present an 80-year-old female who suffered PTSD following exposure to trauma during the triple disaster of the GEJE. The authors noted that her recovery was greatly enhanced by the social support she received while living in Idobata-Nagaya community housing, where residents could naturally discuss their traumatic experiences in a supportive environment (Hori, A., et al., 2018). In another report, Orui and colleagues examined suicide rates in evacuation areas after the Fukushima disaster and found that suicide rates for males increased significantly immediately after the disaster, and then began to increase again 4 years after the disaster. Whereas, female suicide rates declined slightly during the first year after the disaster, but then they increased significantly over the subsequent 3 year period (Orui, M., et al., 2018b).

Looking at the mental health impact of disasters beyond the GEJE, Alfanso (2018) examined suicide rates in Puerto Rico related to Hurricane Maria in 2017 and found that there was an average of 19 suicides per month in the 8 months before Hurricane Maria compared to 25 suicides per month in the 3 months after Maria (32% increase). In another study, Irimpen (2016) reviewed 2,341 medical records for prevalence of various illnesses pre-Hurricane Katrina versus post-Katrina. He reported significant increases in the post-Katrina records, as follows.

-Coronary artery disease	(pre - 30.7% ... post - 47.9%)
-Diabetes	(pre - 28.7% ... post - 39.9%)
-Hypertension	(pre - 74.0% ... post - 80.6%)
-Hyperlipidemia	(pre - 45.0% ... post - 59.3%)
-Smoking	(pre - 39.3% ... post - 53.8%)
-Drug abuse	(pre - 6.7% ... post - 16.4%)
-Psychiatric problems	(pre - 14.9% ... post - 30.7%)

Additionally, the literature documents the impact of displacement on the mental health of those forced to leave their homes due to a disaster. From 2008 to 2015, climate and weather-related disasters displaced an average of 22.5 million people annually. Regardless of the stimulus for migration, recent literature finds some evidence of poorer mental health and wellbeing among migrants and displaced populations relative to populations of non-movers (Torres, J.M. & Casey, J.A., 2017).

In a study examining the mental health impact of displacement, Schwartz et al examined the mental health impact of those displaced by Hurricane Sandy in the New York City area and report that displacement is associated with negative mental health outcomes. Displaced participants were more likely to have PTSD, depression, anxiety symptoms, and increased perceived stress scores as compared to nondisplaced participants (Schwarts, R.M., et al., 2018).

III. Summary and Recommendations

Based on a review of the literature on the mental health impact of natural disasters and reports by respected international agencies, such as, the United Nations and the World Health Organization, natural disasters cause significant impact on the mental health and well-being of those affected. PTSD, depression, anxiety, substance abuse, relationship problems, and suicide are well documented as a result of natural disasters. As such, post-disaster intervention programs need to be prepared to encounter a multitude of mental health problems in the impacted population and thus, programs need to utilize state-of-the-art, evidence based, best practices in addressing the aforementioned problems.

Therefore, the authors have two recommendations. First, it is recommended that a follow up study be conducted to assess the mental health and well-being of those impacted by the GEJE. Second, the authors recommend that a symposium be convened to bring global experts in the area of post-disaster mental health to examine the lessons learned from the GEJE and other global natural disasters, and to develop a plan that could be disseminated globally for addressing the mental health needs of impacted populations.

IV. Conclusion

As stated in the introduction, global disasters are on the rise; thus, the health and mental health impact of disasters are also on the rise. The GEJE triple disaster (earthquake, tsunami, and nuclear disaster) stands as one of the world's major disasters. As we approach the ten year anniversary of the GEJE, it seems prudent that we take time to reflect on the lessons learned from the GEJE and attempt to set a path ahead to improve our response to the mental health impact of such disasters.

References

Alfanso, C.A., 2018. PTSD and Suicide after Natural Disasters. *Psychiatric Times*, 35(4), Available from: http://www.psychiatrictimes.com/ptsd/ptsd-and-suicide-after-natural-disasters [Accessed 24 April 2018]

Centre for Research on the Epidemiology of Disasters, 2017. Annual Disaster Statistical Review 2016 – The numbers and trends. Available from: https://dial.uclouvain.be/pr/boreal/object/boreal%3A190155/datastream/PDF_01/view [Accessed 25 January 2019]

Dai, W., Chen, L., Lai, Z., Wang, J., Liu, A., 2016. The incidence of post-traumatic stress disorder among survivors after earthquakes: a systematic review and meta-analysis. *BMC Psychiatry* 16 (188), doi: 10.1186/s12888-016-0891-9.

Hori, A., Morita, T., Yoshida, I., Tsubokura, M., 2018. Enhancement of PTSD treatment through social support in Idobata-Nagaya community housing after Fukushima's triple disaster. *BMJ Case Rep*, doi:10.1136/bcr-2018-224935.

Irimpen, A., 2016. A rising tide of heart attacks followed Hurricane Katrina, American Heart Association Meeting Report. New Orleans, LA, USA: Available from: https://www.eurekalert.org/pub_releases/2016-11/aha-art110316.php [Public released 15 November 2016]

Ito, S., Sasaki, M., Okabe, S., Konno, N., Goto, A., 2018. Depressive Symptoms and Associated Factors in Female Students in Fukushima Four Years after the Fukushima Nuclear Power Plant Disaster. *International Journal of Environmental Research and Public Health*, 15(11), pii: E2411. doi: 10.3390/ijerph15112411.

Live Science, 2017. Japan Earthquake & Tsunami of 2011: Facts and Information. Live Science, 13 September. Available from: https://www.livescience.com/39110-japan-2011-earthquake-tsunami-facts.html [Accessed 25 January 2019]

Mollica, R.F., Lopes Cardozo, B., Osofsky, H.J., Raphael, B., Ager, A., Salama, P., 2004. Mental health in complex emergencies. *The Lancet*, 364(9450), 2058-67.

Neria, Y., Nandi, A., Galea, S., 2008. Post-traumatic stress disorder following disasters: a systematic review. *Psychological Medicine*, 38(4), 467-480.

Orui, M., Nakajima, S., Takebayashi, Y., Ito, A., Momoi, M., Maeda, M., Yasumura, S., Ohto, H., 2018a. Mental Health Recovery of Evacuees and Residents from the Fukushima Daiichi Nuclear Power Plant Accident after Seven Years - Contribution of Social Network and a Desirable Lifestyle. *International Journal of Environmental Research and Public Health*, 15(11), pii: E2381, doi: 10.3390/ijerph15112381.

Orui, M., Suzuki, Y., Maeda, M., Yasumura, S., 2018b. Suicide Rates in the Evacuation Areas After the Fukushima Daiichi Nuclear Disaster. *Crisis*, 39(5), 353-363, doi: 10.1027/0227-5910/a000509.

Schwartz, R.M., Rasul, R., Kerath, S.M., Watson, A.R., Lieberman-Cribbin, W., Lui, B., Taioli, E., 2018. Displacement during Hurricane Sandy: The impact on mental health. *Journal of Emergency Management*, 16(1), 17-27.

Torres, J.M., Casey, J.A., 2017. The centrality of social ties to climate migration and mental health. *BMC Public Health*, 17 (600), doi: 10.1186/s12889-017-4508-0.

Tsujiuchi, T., Yamaguchi, M., Masuda, K., Tsuchida, M., Inomata, T., Kumano, H., Kikuchi, Y., Augusterfer, E.F., Mollica, R.F., 2016. High Prevalence of Post-Traumatic Stress Symptoms in Relation to Social Factors in Affected Population One Year after the Fukushima Nuclear Disaster. *PLoS One*, 11(3), e0151807, doi:10.1371/journal.pone.0151807.

United Nations High Commissioner on Refugees, 19 June 2018. Global Trends in Forced Displacement, Available from: https://www.alnap.org/help-library/global-trends-forced-displacement-in-2017 [Accessed 25 January 2019]

World Bank Report on Psychosocial Support in Fragile and Conflict-Affected Settings, 9 May 2016. Available from: http://www.worldbank.org/en/topic/fragilityconflictviolence/brief/psychosocial-support-in-fragile-and-conflict-affected-settings [Accessed 25 January 2019]

World Health Organization, 22 March 2018. Depression fact sheet, Available from: https://www.who.int/news-room/fact-sheets/detail/depression [Accessed 25 January 2019]

2 Mental Health / Community Health / Policy Making

Psycho-social Suffering and Structural Violence after the Fukushima Nuclear Disaster

Takuya Tsujiuchi MD, PhD[*1, *2] *(Medical Anthropology)*

Key words: Fukushima nuclear disaster, post-traumatic stress disorder (PTSD), psycho-social suffering, structural violence, social abuse

I. Introduction

As a result of the Great East Japan Earthquake (GEJE) on March 11th, 2011, the Fukushima nuclear disaster occurred. The magnitude 9.0 earthquake and major Tsunami hit the Pacific coast of northeastern Japan causing the meltdown of four reactors of Fukushima Daiichi Nuclear Power Plant from March 12th to 15th with the subsequent distribution of radioactive substances within the exposed area. This disaster has been compared to the Chernobyl Nuclear disaster in 1986 which also measured level 7 on the International Nuclear Event Scale.

The government of Japan declared a nuclear emergency on March 11th, forcing the evacuation of citizens within a 20km radio of the disaster zone on March 12th, and those living between 20 and 30km were urged to evacuate on March 25th. At the time of the evacuation, 80% of the evacuees did not have accurate information regarding the degree of severity of the nuclear accident (Kurokawa, K., 2012). Most of them thought the evacuation would last only for several days, and therefore they only took personal belongings and necessities with them. Later, most of the evacuees learned the details of the disaster from television news, which repeatedly showed the explosion of the first nuclear reactor. This news caused intense fear, horror or helplessness.

The termination declaration of this accident was issued by the Prime Minister of Japan on December 2011. Nonetheless, the radioactive substances were still continu-

---

*1 Professor, Faculty of Human Sciences, Waseda University
*2 Director, Waseda Institute of Medical Anthropology on Disaster Reconstruction (WIMA)

120   Part II - 2

ously leaking into the air and the Pacific Ocean (New York Times, 2013.09.04). Out of 150,000 evacuees from Fukushima prefecture, 90,000 are relocated to another region within Fukushima prefecture, and about 60,000 residents were relocated to other prefectures, such as, Yamagata, Tokyo, Niigata and Saitama.

II. Our Research Outcome on Evacuees and Victims

The authors performed the multi-method studies from the early stages; anthropological field work study, semi-structural interview study, and large-scale questionnaire survey. All these studies are conducted as a "response" to the "call" from the evacuees, victims, parties concerned, supporters, and administrators.

1. Study 1 [March, 2011]: Survey at temporary shelter in Saitama
(Tsujiuchi, T., et al., 2012a)

One week after the earthquake, the Saitama Super Arena, which was normally used as a multipurpose hall for concerts and shows, was converted into a large temporary shelter. More than 2,500 evacuated people lived for about two weeks in the Arena. "Shinsai-Shien-Network Saitama (SSN)", one of the unofficial support groups, conducted a questionnaire survey in order to evaluate the needs of the evacuees. By the analysis of this survey, we determined the target of the support; child-caring generation mother and child and elderly generation.

2. Study 2 [May, 2011]: Qualitative analysis of the free-answer questionnaire by Futaba town (Tsujiuchi, T., et al., 2012b)

Futaba Town in Fukushima Prefecture is located on the coast of the Pacific Ocean called "Hama Avenue", with a population of about 7,000. Two of the six reactors of the failed Fukushima No.1 nuclear power plant are located in Futaba town, and almost all the regions are within 10km of the nuclear plant. On the next day of the earthquake, 2,200 inhabitants of the town were evacuated to Kawamata town, 40km away from the nuclear plant. But as the radiation levels were also ascending at Kawamata, 1,200 inhabitants were evacuated again to Saitama Prefecture which is 200km from the nuclear plant. The functions of the Futaba town were also moved to Saitama Prefecture. Two months after the disaster, the board of education of Futaba Town conducted an opinion survey, and our team was asked to analyze it. The analysis of free-answer questions shows a great number of issues such as "no place to resettle in", "no information about schoolmates", "family members separated", "difficulty in finding employment", "economic matters", and "radioactive contamination". After this survey, the Futaba local government implemented a great number of measures, such as, school children's summer meetings, mail magazine information, and many Futaba's elementary and junior high school teachers got additional posts in Saitama and Fukushima prefectures.

3. Study3 [Oct, 2011 to March, 2013]: Establishment of Public-private Cooperative Systems (Tsujiuchi, T., et al., 2012a)

Seven months after the earthquake, most of the evacuated people left their temporary shelters and settled-in on a long term basis as refugees in their new local community. However, (1) lack of information and lack of social support, and (2) lack of understanding by the local population were problems. Because these two problems were found by several support groups, it was necessary to make public-private cooperative systems to support the evacuated people. As the public groups have personal information and the private groups have the know-how of concrete support, a new support system must be created by the concepts of social inclusion. In Saitama Prefecture, several local governments, professional associations and private support groups gathered by calling from Saitama Bar Association established a liaison committee on earthquake disaster countermeasures.

4. Study4 [Nov, 2011 to Sep, 2014]: Semi-structural interview study of "Trauma Story" narratives (Tsujiuchi, T. & Masuda, K., 2019)

This study was planned from an idea of a disaster victim who said to us "memories of the disaster must not fade away and it is important to remember in the future of Japan". Fifteen informants have been interviewed and we are planning to continue this study to follow up their life and community regeneration. The "trauma story" narratives of evacuees demonstrated the overwhelming trauma and dreadful absurdity of running for shelter. The condition of evacuation was absolutely disastrous which is similar to reports of experiences by refugees from wars or other large global disasters.

5. Study5 [April, 2011 still continuing]: Anthropological field work study as a member of private support group (Tsujiuchi, T. & Masuda, K., 2019)

I have been working as one of the committee members of the private support group, Shinsai-Shien Network Saitama (SSN). I participate by observing several events and social support actions, and I also visit temporary shelters and temporary housings. Our group has been conducting the following five support actions. One, holding a regular consultation program with specialty collaborating psychologists and lawyers, whom victims can consult regarding any kind of trouble and difficulty in daily life. Second, organizing small social community parties and a community coffee room to encourage talking freely over sweets and coffee. Third, making a social solution list, which includes the contact address of local government, public welfare service, free consulting social support groups, medical clinics and hospital, and the address of regional community parties. Forth, publishing a community flyer called "Fuku-Tama" providing information to support daily lives. Fifth, organizing training seminars to encourage the leaders of private support groups to master the skills of psychological listening techniques and social work.

122   Part II - 2

6. Study6 [2012, 2013, 2014, 2015, 2016, 2017]: Large-scale questionnaire survey
(Tsujiuchi, T., et al., 2016a, 2016b, Tsujiuchi, T., 2016, Yamaguchi, M., 2016, Iwagaki, T., 2017)

The first large-scale questionnaire survey (Tsujiuchi, T., et al., 2016a) was held one year after the disaster by our research team in Waseda University and Shinsai-Shien-Network Saitama (SSN). The questionnaires were distributed to 2011 households evacuated to Saitama Prefecture by the cooperation in disaster response headquarters in Fukushima Prefecture. The response rates were 24.4%. Extremely high-level Post Traumatic Stress Symptoms were evaluated. Our surveys have used the internationally validated Impact of Event Scale-Revised (IES-R) to measure the degree of Post-Traumatic Stress Disorder (PTSD). By the IES-R which is the most internationally used measure in the disaster field, and the psychometric validation studies were shown in different cultural contexts. A score of 25 points or more indicates that PTSD is a clinical concern or PTSD possibility, and 30 or more is seen as warranting a clinical diagnosis of PTSD. This survey on March 2012, mean score is 36.3±21.5, and about 67.3% evacuees are over 24/25 cut-off point determined as broadly defined PTSD which means high-risk presence of probable PTSD.

Second large scale survey (Tsujiuchi, T., et al., 2016b) was conducted by our research team jointed with Nihon-Housou-Kyokai (NHK) Japan Broadcasting Corporation two year after the disaster on March 2013. 2,425 households living at temporary housings within Fukushima prefecture were asked to answer the Impact of Event Scale-Revised (IES-R) and the self-report questionnaires that we generated in order to evaluate the damage by the disaster in relation to several bio-psycho-social factors in refugee lives. There were 745 replies, the cooperation rate was 30.7%. High level PTS symptoms were also found. The mean score of IES-R was 34.2±20.6, and 64.6% were over the cut-off point.

Table 1 lists the outcomes of our research over the past six years. On a yearly basis our research in cooperation with SSN gathered all registered evacuees in Saitama and Tokyo. This allows an annual comparison, though in a strict sense it is not a cohort study.

PTSD is a concept included in the DSM-III psychiatric diagnostic classification by the American Psychiatry Association in 1980. It considers the stress disability that arises from life threatening events such as disasters, accidents, war, disputes, and assaults. The concept states '(1) the person experienced, witnessed, or was confronted with an event or events that involved actual or threatened death or serious injury, or a threat to the physical integrity of self or others. (2) The person's response involved intense fear, helplessness, or horror'. In Japan this concept became better known after the Great Hanshin Earthquake of 1995.

Psycho-social Suffering and Structural Violence after the Fukushima Nuclear Disaster   123

PTSD has three types of symptoms. First there are intrusion symptoms such as flash-backs that repeatedly invade one's consciousness, making the body re-experience the symptoms. For example, suddenly in the middle of work, house duties or childcare, victims re-experience the fear they experienced at the time of the tsunami or nuclear disaster. Secondly there are avoidance symptoms, consisting of conscious or uncon-scious evasion of thoughts, feelings and attitudes regarding the events that caused the psychological shock. For example it may involve evading news and information on the nuclear disaster and the radiation, seeking to dissipate the memory of the disaster. Thirdly there are increased arousal symptoms, such as persistent sleeping disorder, frustration and anger, excessive alertness and nervousness. Someone who has experienced a life-threatening event is likely to unconsciously develop an alert-ness and body preparedness to confront a similar life-threatening event. The majority generally recover after three months. Recovery, however, requires an environment of safety and security.

In table 1, 67.3% of the affected people (2012, Saitama survey), 64.6% (2013, Fuku-shima survey), 59.6% (2013, Saitama and Tokyo survey), 57.7% (2014, Saitama and Tokyo survey), 41.0% (2015, all evacuation places in Japan), 37.7% (2016, Fukushima and all evacuation places in Japan), 46.8% (2017, Capital region survey) showed PTSD possibility. So although the percentages have been gradually declining we find that PTSD was still an issue for almost 40% of evacuees, six years on from the disaster.

Table 1. Six years trend of stress level

Date of survey	2012	2013	2013	2014	2015	2016	2017
Evacuation prefecture	Saitama	Fukushima	Saitama, Tokyo	Saitama, Tokyo	All	Fukushima, All	Capital region
Collaborator	SSN	NHK	SSN	SSN	NHK	SSN	SSN
Sample size	2,011	2,425	4,268	3,599	16,686	5,464	10,275
Collecting size	490	745	530	761	2,862	1,012	1,083
Response rate	24.4%	30.7%	12.4%	23.9%	17.2%	18.5%	10.0%
IES-R Mean±SD	36.31 ±21.46	34.20 ±20.55	31.93 ±21.13	31.07 ±21.59	23.44 ±19.01	22.49 ±18.33	26.14 ±20.22
PTSD possibility	67.3%	64.6%	59.6%	57.7%	41.0%	37.7%	46.8%

*SSN; Shinsai-Shien Network Saitama, NHK; Nihon-Hōsō-Kyōkai

By contrast, about four years after the Kobe Earthquake of 1995 which killed 6,434people, PTSD possibility was about 39.5% of temporary housing residents and the mean score of IES-R was 22.5 (Kato, H., 2000). In the 2004 Niigata Chuetsu Earthquake, which killed 68 people, the corresponding level of PTSD at 13 months was about 21% (Naoi, K., 2009) and the mean score of IES-R was 14.3. The level of PTSD is thus noticeably higher for the Fukushima disaster than was found after the two other disasters. In our previous study (Tsujiuchi, T., et al., 2016a), we discussed all the earthquake and tsunami studies by IES-R in these twenty years. For example, Cetin et al. (2005) reported 27.7 mean IES-R score of volunteer rescue workers in the Turkey earthquake of 1999, Wang et al. (2011) reported 26.7 mean IES-R score of refugees collected by psychological relief workstation and local general hospital in the Wenchen Earthquake, China of 2008. Compared to these other disasters around the world, our results the mean score of IES-R from 22.5 to 36.3 indicate relatively higher presence of post-traumatic stress symptoms.

Although there have been few studies evaluated by IES-R since the Fukushima nuclear disaster, Shigemura (2012) found that 30% of workers at the Fukushima No.1 nuclear power plant, where the meltdowns occurred, had IES-R over 25 points when tested two to three months after the disaster, along with 19% of workers at the neighboring No.2 plant. Evacuees of Hirono Town at Fukushima Prefecture showed a 54% rate of PTSD nine months after the disaster (Kukihara, H., et al., 2014). This result is broadly similar to that found in our study. A systematic review of the PTSD research by Yuval Neria (2007) shows the incidence of PTSD after natural disasters ranging from 4 to 60% and after man-made disasters from 5 to 75%, showing that man-made disasters tend to carry higher rates of PTSD. Our research on nuclear disaster, being a human-made disaster, appears to confirm this characteristic trend.

III. Psychological, social and economic factors in post-traumatic stress

Our large scale questionnaire survey makes it statistically clear the considerable influence of the psychological, social and economic factors on post-traumatic stress a multiple logistic regression with IES-R as the objective variable was performed.

The first multiple logistic regression analysis (Tsujiuchi, T., et al., 2016a) of Saitama survey on 2012 is shown in Figure 1. One was "worries about livelihood sustainability" (OR: 2.3), the second was "concerns about yet unsolved issues of compensation and reparation" (OR: 3.7), and the third was "loss of their jobs" (OR: 1.7). The main cause of unemployment was due to displacement and transmigration. Moreover, the subsequent delays of the monetary compensation for the nuclear accident made the economic future uncertain, keeping the stress and social factors related unsolved.

The fourth factor is a "shrinking of human networks and social ties" (OR: 2.3) due to being evacuated and its stigma. The number OR denotes the odd ratio. As an example, 'loss of their jobs' implies a 1.7 times higher risk of having PTSD over those not get loss of their jobs.

The evacuation events destroyed the sustaining bonds between individual and community. Several narratives recorded on free description questions included in our surveys revealed what amount harassment, discrimination and stigma suffered by Fukushima's evacuated residents, is pushing them to hide their real origin within neighborhood.

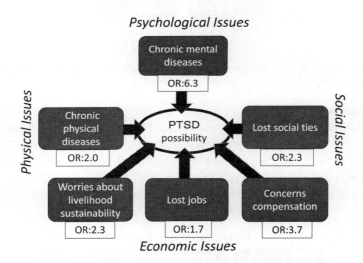

Figure 1. Psychological, social and economic factors affecting the possibility of post-traumatic stress disorder from the Saitama survey on 2012

Second multiple logistic regression analysis (Tsujiuchi, T., et al., 2016b) of Fukushima survey on 2013 is shown in Figure 2. By the result of multiple logistic regression analysis, the significant predictors of PTSD possibility were "economic difficulty" (OR:2.3), "concerns about compensation" (OR:4.2), "aggravation of chronic disease" (OR:2.9), "affection of new disease" (OR:2.2), and "lack of acquaintance support" (OR:1.9).

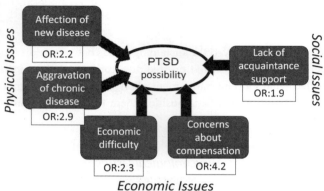

Figure 2. Psychological, social and economic factors affecting the possibility of post-traumatic stress disorder from the Fukushima survey on 2013

Third multiple logistic regression analysis of survey (Tsujiuchi, T., 2016) on 2015 is shown in Figure 3. The significant predictors of PTSD possibility were "fear of dying felt in the first week after the nuclear accident" (OR: 2.0), "worries about livelihood sustainability" (OR: 2.1), "real-estate worries" (OR: 1.4), "worries about loss of hometown" (OR: 1.7), "absence of a reliable other" (OR: 2.0), "unpleasant experiences at evacuation place" (OR: 1.9), and "complaints about family relationships" (OR: 1.9).

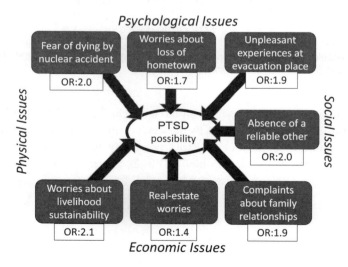

Figure 3. Psychological, social and economic factors affecting the possibility of post-traumatic stress disorder from the survey on 2015

In general, the experiences which tend to cause PTSD are direct violence by war, terrorism, disaster, serious accident, torture, abduction, being taken hostage, physical assault, rape, abuse, or domestic violence (American Psychiatric Association 2013). But in the case of child abuse, not only physical abuse but also repeated complexity of psychological and socio-economic violence became severe traumatic experiences (Herman, J.L., 2015). Considering our result of Fukushima disaster which shows the statistical relationship between several psycho-social economic factors and the possibility of PTSD, it is argued that indirect violence after human-made disaster may also induce PTSD.

IV. Structural violence in Fukushima victims

My analysis of the treatment of nuclear disaster victims matches the concept of structural violence through injustice, inequity, disparity, and discrimination. 'Structural violence' is a term coined by Johan Galtung (1969), the founder of Peace Research. It is a well-known term in the field of global health. In contrast to direct violence exerted by an individual human being, 'structural violence' refers to the indirect violence wrought by the social system and social structure. Structural violence is integrated in the political, economic, social, and cultural structure, and shows up as inequity in power relationships, social injustice, and in daily life as instances of inequity, disparity, and discrimination. Paul Farmer (1997, 2003, 2011), analyzes in detail the abuse and structural violence in poverty and health inequality in Haiti. Farmer (1997) described AIDS and political violence as the two leading causes of death among young adults in Haiti. Bureaucrats and soldiers had unconstrained sway over the lives of the rural poor. These are determined the victims of structural violence by Farmer.

The violence of nuclear disaster undermined deprivation of the roots of 'living conditions, life, and environment'. Moreover, the subsequent setting of policies of 'returning plan to homeland excluding residents' approval' and also 'compensation disparity' became a continuation of structural violence, as it would be an outrage against the daily lives of the victims. However, this phenomenon is only the upper part of the structure. In the substructure are the postwar economic policies promoting the development of nuclear generation of electricity, the inequity of wealth distribution generated by preferential economic measures for big corporations, the structural geopolitical exploitation of antagonism between 'center' and 'countryside', the structure of social disparity based on competition lead by neo-liberalism, the rejection of social responsibility implied by the self-responsibility (jiko sekinin) theory of medical and social services, and the postwar use of National Security as a justification for peaceful use of nuclear energy. The author suggests this is the multilayer structure underlying structural violence in Fukushima.

Next, I will discuss the dimension of mental wounding or trauma and violence. The experience of trauma from various kinds of violence is the cause of PTSD. As I mentioned before, generally PTSD is assumed to stem from physical violence, usually directly inflicted by individuals. Nonetheless, as our research clarifies, the possibility of PTSD has psychological, social and economic influences. Therefore the concept of structural violence at the root of PTSD may be discerned.

Examples of abuse include physical abuse, sexual abuse, psychological abuse, neglect, economic abuse and social abuse. "Social abuse" usually used being dismissed from society, neglected, isolated, and hindered from social participation and activities (Kassah, A.K., 2012). Social system abuse is the lack of access to public services such as medical and social services and pensions, due to neglect by the administration. Furthermore in a broad sense social abuse includes all the poor conditions of life, such as discrimination, poverty and discord, due to faults in the prevalent ideology. Yamano (2009) used the word 'social abuse' in his pathological analysis of societies with sustained child abuse. Yamano criticized the tendentious positioning of psychologism over the pathology of families with child abuse. Rather he pointed to violations of children's human rights due to inadequate budgets for family social services; also due to inadequate social services and education for children, leading to isolation, fragmentation and delay in providing child-care.

After flare-ups of domestic violence, the perpetrators often express their regret. The victims, despite having been beaten and kicked, become dependent on this apologetic attitude and the accompanying words 'I love you'. They cannot get out of this distorted dependent relationship, to the point they come to blame themselves for angering the perpetrator. In this way, the authority, supremacy and power of the perpetrators exerts control over the life and living of victims. Victims subjected to repeated physical and psychological abuse with threats, intimidation, and actual violence, reach a state of resignation, which gradually leads to physical and mental exhaustion, followed in turn by social isolation.

The same applies, structurally speaking, to nuclear disaster damage. There are symbolic similarities between domestic violence and social abuse within the victims of Fukushima disaster. The perpetrators pay consolation money as a symbolic apology and admission of blame. Many politicians, including Prime Minister Shinzō Abe, have stated: 'There can be no revival of Japan without the recovery of Fukushima'. These words mean symbolically "I love Fukushima". But deep down, contrary to these words, issues such as radiation contamination and the continuing nuclear disaster remain segregated as 'Fukushima problems'. These problems are not only limited to Fukushima but also to other regions.

Psycho-social Suffering and Structural Violence after the Fukushima Nuclear Disaster   129

Again, politicians and national government officials express apologies by saying 'We regret the forced evacuation', but will seek to break down the resistance of residents by cancelling the evacuation order. 'It is safe, and secure, it is all clear' – they repeat these sweet words along with the domestic discourse on the 'myth of safety and security (*Anzen Anshin Shinwa*)', pressurizing residents to return to yet land whose safety is not yet assured. Meanwhile, due to their great economic losses, the victims cannot rebuild their lives. They need compensation money from TEPCO and national government. Some voluntary evacuees have come to blame their predicament on their own selfish refusal to return to Fukushima. Physically and mentally they have become exhausted. Due to unpleasant experiences at their places of evacuation destination, they have hidden their identities as refugees, and have been driven into social isolation. In this way victims are been deprived of their right to make their own life decisions. Indeed, it can be said that this is 'social abuse'.

V. Social abuse cases due to structural violence

In this section, I will demonstrate five written statements from the free writing space provided in the 2015 questionnaire. From 563 respondents in the free writing section, 48 cases with rich narratives and full descriptions were selected, using the key words "death" or "dying" to evaluate seriousness, and five cases were determined to be typical cases of social abuse. One other purpose of presenting these cases is to illustrate collective psycho-social and economic suffering, as described in the quantitative analysis section. At the top of each case report, the results of stress level (IES-R) and the seven items of psycho-social and economic factors thought to influence PTSD possibility are shown.

1. Case 1 (ID.445: Compulsory evacuee)
IES-R=47, fear of dying by nuclear disaster (-), worries about loss of hometown (++), Unpleasant experiences at evacuation place (-), absence of a reliable other (+), complaints about family relationships (+), real-estate worries (+), worries about livelihood sustainability (+).

67 y.o. female, evacuated from Futaba town, Fukushima prefecture to Soka city, Saitama Prefecture; living in a very cramped room with her 90 y.o father and 85 y.o. mother. She herself needing nursing care is compelled to provide her elderly parents' nursing care. Her father is used to sitting all day at the kotatsu (a Japanese low covered table with a heat source) and her mother after sweeping the apartment in the early morning sleeps inside it.

'No one is expected to visit, there is no place to go, and we just eat three times a day and sleep. There is nothing to do'.

130   Part II - 2

Society has rejected and neglected them, isolated them, and their social participation and activities are disabled. Indeed this condition is 'social abuse'.

'Actually this condition is as distressing as dying. We understand the feelings of those who committed suicide. But dying is easy. Those being released of pain by death may go in peace, yet for those who remain, without a clear future and without the possibility of dying, there is only pain. It is better to live and share the adversity together. However the truth is, it is as hard as dying'.

Moreover, though they are not permitted to return to their hometown, with their actual savings they cannot afford to buy land and house, and are obliged to continue the desperate struggle of their evacuees' life.

'We can't go back. My parents are 90 and 85. I feel awful, we don't have any permanent settlement, we are condemned to wait for death without any hope. Our actual savings don't allow us to buy a home. I wish we could live in a small apartment building but TEPCO does not cover the cost of buying a family home. It is better for families with elderly and disabled ones living conditions to live in apartment buildings near train and bus stations, near hospitals. My husband worked for TEPCO, that is why we don't like to complain to TEPCO. I have heard that those who moved to Iwaki city have built fine houses, yet they are not-well considered by local people in Iwaki. Those were people who were already rich, and they quickly settled down in Iwaki. Common people like us can't do the same. Therefore, our future is uncertain'.

The previous account explains how the policy of compensation and indemnity after the nuclear disaster itself works out as structural violence, dominating the life and living conditions of the victims.

2. Case 2 (ID.1274: Compulsory evacuee)

IES-R=61, fear of dying by nuclear disaster (-), worries about loss of hometown (++), unpleasant experiences at evacuation place (++), absence of a reliable other (-), complaints about family relationships (-), real-estate worries (+), worries about livelihood sustainability (+).

37 y.o. female, evacuated from Futaba Town, Fukushima prefecture to Iwaki city, in the southern part of the same prefecture. She had divorced just before the disaster and became an evacuee with her daughter and son. Due to the deep psychological pressure she had a suicidal inclination. Several times she thought of returning to their hometown in Futaba and committing suicide there.

'I would like to die. I would like to be killed. There is no sense of living in my

Psycho-social Suffering and Structural Violence after the Fukushima Nuclear Disaster   131

life, rather I am thinking of organ donation. In any case I would like to disap-
pear. I understand the feelings of longing for suicide. I myself thought of going
back to Futaba and committing suicide... then my children's face appear... I
can't... next year my elder daughter will be a high school student... it is enough,
please allow me to die.'

She cannot have her parents' support as her old mother is living alone elsewhere in
Fukushima prefecture far from Iwaki city. When she got divorced, her former husband gave her the family house in lieu child support payments. However, the nuclear
disaster and radioactive contamination made the house uninhabitable. Her former
husband received financial compensation, and since then has been evading her.

'I got divorced one month before the disaster. Instead of the monetary support
for raising our children I remained living at the house, which was still in his
name, because there were still loan payments to make that he said he would
take care of. He promised that after the loan payment was completed he would
formally transfer the property to our son. Since he received the compensation
money I have not heard from him, he is evading me. I told this to TEPCO, to the
lawyer, and they just said that sometimes this happens...I would like them to
think about measures to deal with this.'

'My two children are much stressed. They stopped attending school. My oldest
daughter kicked and broke down the wall of our rented house with her emotional instability. This rebellious age is very hard to cope with, it due to her
psychological state. For several reasons it is so uncomfortable, I feel too emotionally unstable to raise my children, nor can I go out to work... it hurts me
psychologically. I don't want to go out.'

As we see here, the stormy psychological state she had fallen into is setting up originally by domestic violence from her divorced husband. The violence includes emotional abuse, economic abuse, using male privilege, using children, and isolation. The
nuclear disaster excessively intensify her damages by this violence.

She wrote about the harassment she gets from the neighborhood. It is not only harassment in their neighborhood but also at work. When they knew her evacuee status it
became in such a poor work environment, that until now she is not able to work.

'Before the disaster we lived in a detached house. Now it is difficult to adjust to
the noisy living in an apartment. Moreover I dislike the word 'evacuee'. It is
easy to get harassment. I came here (Iwaki City), and worked nights, part-time
at Family Mart. I did it so I could look after my children during the day-time. I

132   Part II - 2

do receive compensation money. Though I was struggling just to get by, they would say 'Treat me to dinner!' 'You are getting rich!' I got this kind of verbal harassment at work, countless stupid words, so I quit. Since then I've been afraid to work, I can't work'.

In addition to the physiological and economic violence from her former husband, the extremely hard social abuse she experienced put her in a very dangerous state.

3. Case 3 (ID.174: Formerly compulsory evacuee, but now voluntary evacuee)

IES-R=34, fear of dying by nuclear disaster (-), worries about loss of hometown (-), unpleasant experiences at evacuation place (++), absence of a reliable other (+), complaints about family relationships (-), real-estate worries (+), worries about livelihood sustainability (no answer).

67-year-old female, evacuated from Hirono town, Fukushima prefecture to Iwaki City in the same prefecture. She has high blood pressure and has had a cerebral infarction. The evacuation order for Hirono was lifted six months after the nuclear disaster; those not returning to their hometown were reclassified as 'voluntary evacuees'. One year after the imposition of the evacuation order by the government, none of the Hirono residences had received compensation from TEPCO. Through the mere fact of becoming evacuees, they have received an intense, visible kind of social violence from the neighborhood. It is not difficult to imagine the psychological suffering resulting from these conditions.

'I have been harassed many times by unknown neighbors. Dead snakes and toads are left at my front door. We notified the police and the patrol car came. Some old people shouts insults to me 'Drop dead, you old hag!' (Shine, kusobaba). There are a lot of lonely elderly people around here, and there are no social activities organized in neighborhood. I am scared of anonymous strange men living next to me'.

She feels afraid of her unfamiliar neighbors to the point where her life might be at risk, because she thinks no-one is bothered about abusive acts, and if nothing is done these acts will increase. She is considered to be a rich evacuee compensated by TEPCO, and has become an object of envy to her neighbors. Social isolation is resulting from the insecure living conditions of evacuees.

4. Case 4 (ID.620: Voluntary evacuee)

IES-R=28, fear of dying by nuclear disaster (-), worries about loss of hometown (++), unpleasant experiences at evacuation place (-), absence of a reliable other (+), complaints about family relationships (+), real-estate worries (-), worries about livelihood sustainability (+).

Psycho-social Suffering and Structural Violence after the Fukushima Nuclear Disaster   133

36 y.o. male evacuated from Koriyama city, Fukushima prefecture to Aomori city, Aomori prefecture. He is a so-called 'voluntary evacuee'. The following quotation is his account of the suffering of one of his relatives that committed suicide after getting divorced.

> 'I understand very well the feelings of those who committed suicide. I've been one step away from doing the same thing. My cousin committed suicide one year and a few months ago. Like me, he became an evacuee because of the nuclear accident; later he got divorced and in the end he committed suicide. His memorial photo reminds me of myself. We had no choice. Even now I hate TEPCO. TEPCO has committed manslaughter.'

This statement shows the cruelty of the conditions of social violence leading to commit suicide. The narrator himself suffered from depression after the nuclear disaster, and is still undergoing treatment. 'It is tough. Some days I feel down, some days I feel irritated,' he complained. His irritation was prompted by the persistent propaganda of the central government and Fukushima Prefecture about the safety and security of districts having their evacuation orders lifted, in spite of lingering contamination levels that he sees as preventing the safe raising of children.

> 'Again and again they say it is safe, it is secure, yet until the conditions for safely raising children are reached, their words are meaningless. I want to go back to a safe hometown'.

Moreover 'There is antagonism in my family over evacuation and the future. I feel helpless'. Finally, he expressed his consent over the future of his country.

> 'Somehow or other we have to go back to the state before the nuclear accident. Therefore at least, we expect the authorities to take responsibility and provide compensation. Japan's constitution assures preeminent respect for the human person, not for the business company or the country. Nonetheless, Japan is protecting TEPCO and the country above the human person. It is a deplorable situation; I am worried about the future of such a Japan'.

5. Case 5 (ID.1427: Voluntary evacuee)
IES-R=62, fear of dying by nuclear disaster (+), worries about loss of hometown (-), unpleasant experiences at evacuation place (-), absence of a reliable other (+), complaints about family relationships (++), real-estate worries (-), worries about livelihood sustainability (+).

38 y.o. female evacuated from Koriyama city, Fukushima prefecture to Hiroshima prefecture. She is a so-called 'voluntary evacuee'. Her husband remained in Fuku-

shima prefecture in order not to lose his job and income. The following narrative is her account of suffering as a 'mother and child evacuee'.

> 'I have a four-year-old son. When the earthquake and nuclear accident occurred, he was only one. From that time, it has been the same as having no father. She cannot remember her father's face. Really, it is too far from Hiroshima to Fukushima. So, coming and going is so tough. My husband is living alone in Fukushima and becoming nasty dissolute and despondent. I don't know what his life is really like. Along with the long distance, it is difficult to communicate with each other. Love and affection have already gone.'

This serious family split was caused by the nuclear disaster. This is not a special case. A lot of 'nuclear disaster divorce cases' (*genpatsu rikon*) have been reported by supporters of the victims. In the background to this division lie differing assessment of radiation risk. Most voluntary evacuees, particularly women, are acutely concerned about the danger of low dose radiation contamination, especially for babies and children. Their decision to escape from Fukushima was often based on careful gathering of information on radiation and health issues. In contrast, many male or elderly people, already disinclined to leave their homeland dues to economic concerns or wishing to maintain local human networks, believe the government's safety assurances – the so called '*anzen-anshin shinwa*' or 'myth of safety and security'.

> 'It is tough. I never rest. Every day, I have to work hard to get income and of course I have to take care of my child. My body is falling apart, I am on the verge of collapse. I fear I may not live to see my son grow up. The rent is expensive. I really don't have enough money. I heard that some of my acquaintances have been forced into working at sex industry.'

She is also troubled about her livelihood. Because of her double life between Fukushima and Hiroshima, she has to maintain two households.

6. Case Discussion
All these five cases may be understood as victims of structural violence. Galtung (1969) described structural violence as being built into the structure and showing up as unequal power and consequently as unequal life chances. Indeed, all the people in the case studies were deprived of life chances and thrown into a tragic life. If there had been no nuclear accident, they could have continued their own normal lives and their fundamental human rights would not have been violated. Along with this definition by Galtung, it is necessary to evaluate the system or structure of indirect violence. Farmer (1997) described the national or international mechanisms that create and deepen inequalities and which are part of the system of structural violence.

In our Fukushima study, I evaluated the complex socio-economic and political system of structural violence (Figure 4). Two aspects of main structural violence are determined. One is the setting of evacuation and return orders without reference to an appropriate radiation dose, and the second is the discourse known as the 'myth of safety and security' (*Anzen Anshin Shinwa*). From these kinds of violence, widening disparity in compensation between compulsory evacuees and voluntary evacuees, and the division of local communities have emerged.

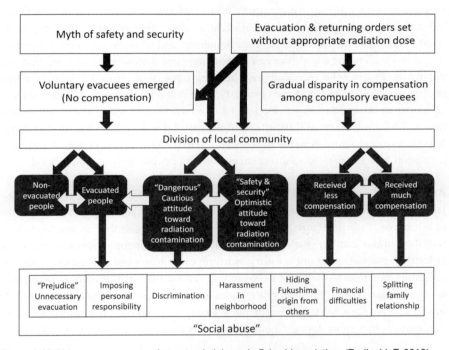

Figure 4. Multi-layer components of structural violence in Fukushima victims (Tsujiuchi, T. 2019)

The evacuation orders imposed and then sometimes lifted by the Japanese government may be read as a kind of main political violence. Anand Grover, special rapporteur to the United Nations Human Rights Council, called on the government of Japan to 'formulate a national plan on evacuation zones and dose limits of radiation by using current scientific evidence, based on human rights rather than on a risk-benefit analysis, and reduce the radiation dose to less than 1mSv/year' (Grover A. 2012). The World Health Organization has also analyzed the health risk after the Fukushima Nuclear Accident using dose-response relationship scientific theory (WHO 2013). Without reference to these recommendations by an international agency, the Japanese government chose 20mSv/year as the borderline dose for lifting evacuation orders. This government's decision was not based on appropriate scientific evidence (CSRP 2016). Although the Japanese government is not the direct perpetrator of violence, it is part of the system which creates inequity, disparity, and discrimination affecting victims. Because of the government's evacuation order, voluntary evacuees emerged. If there had been different criteria such as 1mSv/year, fewer voluntary evacuees would have appeared.

Since unequal compensation payments resulted from the enforcing and lifting of evacuation orders, the local community was divided into several groups experiencing different damages and benefits, leading to envy, discrimination and neighborhood feuds over who can return to their homeland and who can get more compensation. Even just among compulsory evacuees, there are obvious gaps in compensation payments. People who own land and housing have done relatively well, whereas people who don't have their own property have fallen into poverty. We can observe 'disparity in compensation' in case 1 and 2 in which victims received less compensation and fell into 'financial difficulties'. In the case 3, the invisible structural violence of prejudice, stemming from the misconception that all the evacuees got a lot of compensation, was manifested as direct harassment by people in the neighborhood.

Another kind of social violence stems from the 'myth of safety and security'. The Japanese government (the Cabinet Office, Reconstruction Agency, and the Ministry of Education, Culture, Sports, Science and Technology) insists that an annual dose of radiation under 20mSv/year is safe. Believing this myth, people have come to view voluntary evacuation as unnecessary, wanting to impose personal responsibility on voluntary evacuees to make their own living. The cautious attitude toward radiation contamination taken by voluntary evacuees is regarded as 'radiation phobia', resulting in serious cases of prejudice of unnecessary evacuation', 'discrimination' and 'harassment in neighborhoods' against voluntary evacuees, as seen in cases 4 and 5.

Farmer (1997) discussed multiaxial models of suffering. The axis of gender is one of the important issues of structural violence. He notes that men have dominated political, legal, and economic institutions to varying degrees in every society. Joshua M. Price (2012) also analyzed the hidden brutality in the lives of women. In cases 2 and 5, gender inequality is an evident factor. In case 2, the victim asked a lawyer to save the situation, but learned that there are no legal protection. Serious splits in family relationship's led these victims into 'nuclear power plant divorce' (genpatsu rikon), and the stress of child care seems to have been a severe psychological stress factor. The results of the IES-R score are extremely high at over 60 points in these two cases.

As I mentioned earlier in this paper, a score of 25 points or more in IES-R indicates that PTSD is a clinical possibility, and 30 or more is seen as warranting a clinical diagnosis of PTSD. The IES-R score of case 1 is 47, case 2 is 61, case 3 is 34, case 4 is 28, and case 5 is 62. Serious psychological problems are revealed by these scores. As I indicated in the introduction to each case, more than three items of psycho-social and economic risks of quantitative data were found in every case. According to each case's qualitative data, collective psycho-social and economic difficulties were also discovered, and multi-layer components of structural violence can be observed.

VI. Acute-on-chronic: pathological social structure

From our quantitative and qualitative analysis, 'evacuation and returning orders set without appropriate radiation dose' and the 'myth of safety and security (*Anzen Anshin Shinwa*)' are analyzed as distinct cases of structural violence. However, these phenomena are only part of the superstructure. Farmer (2011), analyzing the acute social problems after the Haiti earthquake, realized that there are chronic social disabilities engendered over five centuries by transnational social and economic forces with deep roots in the colonial enterprise. Following Farmer's work, we can argue that a 'pathological chronic state', in other words 'basic structural violence', were also factors in the Fukushima disaster.

First, postwar economic policies promoting the development of nuclear generation of electricity, and postwar use of 'national security' as a justification for peaceful use of nuclear energy are important. Fujigaki (2015) indicated the historical process through which nuclear power plants are embedded in the political, economic, and social context in Japan. Fujigaki described also the way of cultural acceptance of nuclear energy. Japan is the only country ever to have experienced atomic bombing, and people have a strong fear that nuclear energy may kill civilians. However, Fujigaki noticed various policies promoting 'atoms for peace' appealing to tropes of 'autonomy', 'openness' and 'democratic control'. This history made the 'myth of safety and security' part of the superstructure of structural violence.

Second, the structure of social disparity based on competition led by neo-liberalism, the inequity of wealth distribution generated by preferential economic measures for large corporations, and the structural geopolitical exploitation of antagonism between 'center' and 'countryside', along with the rejection of social responsibility implied by the stress on self-responsibility (*jiko sekinin*) by the medical and social services, can be observed. Farmer (2005) criticized this neoliberalism, which generally refers to an ideology advocating the dominance of a competition-driven market model, without caring about the social and economic inequalities that distort real economies. Farmer pointed out that neoliberal policies and ideologies have generally called for the subjugation of political and social life in Latin America.

A similar phenomenon developed in postwar Japan. Takahashi (2012) analyzed the common factors between Fukushima and Okinawa, where US armed forces permanently stay for pan-pacific and national security. Takahashi described this antagonism between the urban center and rural periphery as a 'sacrificial social system'. The central political system put priority on economic development and national security before rural sustainability. Takahashi analyzed this sacrificial system by the logic of historical colonialism. Local social systems and local people are always sacrificed by this colonial rule.

The above ideologies of neoliberalism also erode equality of medical and social services. Tsujiuchi (2012) reported social risk of the discourse on Metabolic Syndrome in Japan from the viewpoint of critical medical anthropology. The concept of Metabolic Syndrome is one of the major medical policies by the national government, which recommends self-control health care and finally demands self-responsibility (*jiko sekinin*) for people's own health status. Thus, health disparity in Japan is formulated by the above ideologies and policies of neoliberalism.

Hence, these several forms of structural violence are the basis of the misfortune brought to the local population by the Fukushima nuclear disaster. Multi-layer components of social forces led directly and indirectly to personal distress.

VII. Conclusion

According to the results of our multi-method studies, anthropological field work study, semi-structural interview, and large-scale questionnaire survey, the current major issues encountered by the evacuees are the complexity of physical, psychological, social, economic, and political problems.

A high level of stress, indicating PTSD possibility, was found almost 40% of the respondents over seven years. The statistical analysis found high levels of stress in evacuees linked to physical factors such as "aggravation of chronic disease, affection of new disease", psychological factors such as "trauma of nuclear disaster, loss of hometown, unpleasant experiences at place of evacuation", and also social factors such as "shrinking of human networks and social ties, lack of acquaintance support, absence of a reliable other, complaints about family relationships", and economic factors such as "loss of their jobs, worries over livelihood sustainability, concerns about yet unsolved issues of compensation and reparation, and worries about real-estate", therefore clarifying the complex interaction of factors.

The analysis of these circumstances of the victims of the nuclear accident indicates the presence of 'social abuse by structural violence'. Social abuse is immersed in the

Psycho-social Suffering and Structural Violence after the Fukushima Nuclear Disaster   139

political, economic, social and cultural structure and emerges as social inequity, unequal social opportunities, disparity and discrimination. The structural violence of the nuclear disaster destroyed the living environment and was exacerbated by government policies of return and compensation. Furthermore, traumatic experiences at the living evacuation places and the need to hide their evacuee status hindered victims from integrating into social activities, leading to neglect, isolation and social exclusion. This state may justifiably be called 'social abuse'. Neglect these psychological, social and economic problems is an affront to social justice.

To overcome the abuse of nuclear disaster victims through structural violence, it is necessary to unpack the social pathology rooted in Japanese society. Violence must not be ignored as if it were somebody else's problem; robust policies on domestic violence and abuse are essential. The assessment of the situation of the victims in this survey finds structural violence on the surface of individual problems, and in the background, imbuing a pathological social structure. The responsibility for this structural violence should be shared by all of us, since we are positioned as an important part of the social structure. Violence is not an issue of the other: it is a pathology nesting right under our feet, one that we dismiss at our peril.

The responsibility of the disaster is still uncertain. The evacuees' psychological and social sufferings simultaneously involve health, welfare, legal, political, economic, and moral issues. It is apparent that, they were injured and inflicted by the social forces. The mental health problems reported by the victims are not individual or personal in their origin, but rather, they should be understood as a context of social responsibility to the disaster; thus fitting the description of post-traumatic stress disorder.

Our findings suggest that it is most important to resolve the various social issues caused by structural violence in order to decrease the psychological stresses impacting the health and mental health of the victims.

Acknowledgements

The author would like to express my sincere gratitude to all the victims reflected in our multiple survey, all the members of the private support team "Shinsai-Shien Network Saitama (SSN)", and the co-researchers and graduate students of the "Waseda Institute of Medical Anthropology on Disaster Reconstruction (WIMA)". The author also appreciate the appropriate advice and supervision from Eugene F. Augusterfer and Richard F. Mollica at Harvard Program in Refugee Trauma (HPRT), Professor Yasushi Kikuchi and Dr Marisa Tsuchida at Waseda University, and Professor Tom Gill at Meiji Gakuin University.

Funding

This work was supported by the grant of 'Japan Society for the Promotion of Science KAKENHI' number 25460915 and 16K09264.

References

American Psychiatric Association, 2013. Diagnostic and statistical manual of mental disorders; fifth edition. Arlington, VA: American Psychiatric Publishing Inc., pp. 265-290.

Cetin, M., Kose, S., Ebrinc, S., et al., 2005. Identification and posttraumatic stress disorder symptoms in rescue workers in the Marmara, Turkey, earthquake. *Journal of Traumatic Stress*, 18, 485-489.

Citizen-Scientist International Symposium on Radiation Protection (CSRP), 2016. The Nihonmatsu Declaration on the Risks of Exposure to Low Doses of Ionising Radiation — A statement by participants to the 6th Citizen Scientist International Symposium on Radiation Protection (7–10 October 2016) in Nihonmatsu, Japan. Availabel from: https://drive.google.com/file/d/0BytLTOi-FEmhN3 lTUzMwVFNielU/view [Accessed 30 April 2018]

Farmer, P., 1997. On suffering and structural violence: A view from below. In: Arthur Kleinman, Veena Das, and Margaret Lock (Eds.), Social Suffering. Berkeley and Los Angeles, California: University of California Press, pp. 261-283.

Farmer, P., 2003. Pathologies of Power: Health, Human Rights, and the New War on the Poor. Berkeley and Los Angeles, California: University of California Press.

Farmer, P., 2011. Haiti After the Earthquake. New York: Public Affairs.

Fujigaki, Y., 2015. The processes through wich nuclear power plants are embedded in political, economic, and social context in Japan. In: Fujigaki, Y. (Eds.), Lessons From Fukushima – Japanese Case Studies on Science, Technology and Society. Switzerland: Springer International Publishing, pp. 7-25.

Galtung, J., 1969. Violence, Peace, and Peace Research. *Journal of Peace Research*, 6 (3), 167-191.

Grover, A., 2012. Report of the Special Rapporteur on the right of everyone to the enjoyment of the highest attainable standard of physical and mental health, Anand Grover, Mission to Japan. Human rights council, twenty-third session, agenda item 3. Available from: https://www.save-children-from-radiation. org/2013/05/24/un-special-rapporteur-anand-grover-s-report-on-fukushima-accident-is-published/ A-HRC-23-41-Add3_en.pdf [Accessed 8 Jun 2017]

Herman, J.L., 2015. Trauma and Recovery: The Aftermath of Violence---From Domestic Abuse to Political Terror. New York, Basic Books.

Iwagaki, T., Tsujiuchi, T., Masuda, K., et al., 2017. Relationships between Individual Social Capital and Mental Health in Elderly People who Left the Prefecture Due to the Fukushima Nuclear Power Plant Disaster. *Japanese Journal of Psychosomatic Medicine*, 57 (2), 173-184.

Kassah, Alexander K., Kassah, Bente L.L., and Agbota, Tete, K., 2012. Abuse of disabled children in Ghana. *Disability & Society*, 27 (5), 689-701.

Kato, H., Iwai, K., 2000. Posttraumatic stress disorder after the Great Hanshin-Awaji

Earthquake—assessment by the structured interview to the survivors. *Medical Journal of Kobe University*, 60, 27-35.

Kukihara, H., Yamawaki, N., Uchiyama K., et al., 2014. Trauma, depression, and resilience of earthquake / tsunami / nuclear disaster survivors of Hirono, Fukushima, Japan. *Psychiatry and Clinical Neurosciences*, 68, 524-533.

Kurokawa, K., Oshima, K., Sakiyama, H., et al., 2012. The official report of the Fukushima nuclear accident independent investigation commission: Executive summary. Tokyo, JAPAN: The National Diet of Japan. pp38-41, Available from: http://warp.da.ndl.go.jp/info:ndljp/pid/3856371/naiic.go.jp/report/

Naoi, K., 2009. Local mental health activity after the Niigata-ken Chuetsu Earthquake: Findings of investigations performed three and half months and thirteen months after the earthquake, and analysis about the risk factor of PTSD. *JPN Bulletin of Social Psychiatry*, 18, 52-62.

Neria, Y., Nandi, A., Galea, S., 2007. Post-traumatic stress disorder following disasters: a systematic review. *Psychological Medicine*, 38, 467-480.

New York Times, September 4, 2013. Errors cast doubt on Japan's cleanup of nuclear accident site. Available from: http://www.nytimes.com/2013/09/04/world/asia/errors-cast-doubt-on-japans-cleanup-of-nuclear-accident-site.html [Accessed 16 April 2014]

Price, J.M., 2012. Structural violence: Hidden brutality in the lives of women. Albany: State University of New York Press.

Shigemura, J., Tanigawa, T., Saito I., et al., 2012. Psychological distress in workers at the Fukushima nuclear power plant. *JAMA*, 308 (7), 667-669.

Takahashi, T., 2012. *Gisei no shisutemu – Fukusima, Okinawa.* [A System of Scapegoats — Fukushima and Okinawa (provisional translation).], Tokyo: Shūeisha.

Tsujiuchi, T., Masuda, K., Chida, Y., Nagatomo, H., Ito, Y., Nakagami, A., Suzuki, K., Inomata, T., 2012a. Establishment of Public-private Cooperative Systems to Support Evacuees from the Nuclear Contaminated Area; A case in Saitama Prefecture. *Jpn J Psychosom Int Med*, 16(2), 261-268.

Tsujiuchi, T., Masuda, K., Nagamoto, H., Chida, Y., Yamashita, S., Yamaguchi, M., Nagumo, S., Awano, S., Ito, Y., Nakagami, A., Suzuki, K., Sato, S., Idogawa, K., 2012b. The Study of Long–term Support to Evacuees from the Disaster of Fukushima Nuclear Power Plant ; Qualitative Analysis of the Survey conducted by the Board of Education of Futaba Town in Fukushima prefecture and Memoir of Victims. *WASEDA Human Sciences*, 25(2), pp273-284.

Tsujiuchi, T., 2012. Social risk of the discourse on Metabolic Syndrome (2nd Report); Analysis of the social responses from the viewpoint of critical medical anthropology. *Japanese Journal of Psychosomatic Medicine*, 52 (10), 927-936.

Tsujiuchi, T., Yamaguchi, M., Masuda, K., Marisa T., Tadashi I., Hiroaki K., Yasushi K., Augusterfer, E.F., Mollica, R.F., 2016a. High prevalence of post-traumatic stress symptoms in relation to social factors in affected population one year after the

Fukushima nuclear disaster. *PLoS ONE*, 11(3), e0151807. doi:10.1371/journal. pone.0151807.

Tsujiuchi, T., Komaki, K., Iwagaki, T., Masuda, K., Yamaguchi, M., Fukuda, C., Ishikawa, N., Mochida, R., Kojima, T., Negayama, K., Ogihara, J., Kumano, H., 2016b. High-level post-traumatic stress symptoms of the residents in Fukushima temporary housing: Bio-psycho-social impacts by nuclear power plant disaster. *Japanese Journal of Psychosomatic Medicine*, 56 (7), 723-736.

Tsujiuchi, T., 2016. *Genpatsu jiko ga motarashita seishinteki higai: kōzō teki bōryoku ni yoru shakaiteki gyakutai.* [Mental health impact of the nuclear accident: Social abuse caused by structural violence.], *Kagaku*, 86 (3), 246-251.

Tsujiuchi, T., 2019. Post-traumatic Stress Due to Structural Violence after Fukushima Disaster. *Japan Forum*: doi:10.1080/09555803.2018.1552308.

Tsujiuchi, T., Masuda K., 2019. *Fukushima no iryō jinrui gaku.* [Medical Anthropology of Fukushima.], Tōmi Shobō.

Yamaguchi, M., Tsujiuchi, T., Masuda, K., Iwagaki, T., Ishikawa, N., Fukuda, C., Hirata, S., Inomata, T., Negayama, K., Kojima, T., Ogihara, J., Kumano, H., 2016. Social Factors Affecting Psychological Stress of the Evacuees Out of Fukushima Prefecture by the Cause of Nuclear Accident after the Great East Japan Earthquake. *Japanese Journal of Psychosomatic Medicine* 56, (8), 819-832.

Yamano, R., 2009. *Shakaiteki gyakutai-ron josetsu.* [Introduction of social abuse.], *Sōgō Shakai Fukushi Kenkyū* (Critical social welfare), 35, 55-63.

Wang, L., Zhang, J., Shi, Z., et al., 2011. Confirmatory factor analysis of posttraumatic stress symptoms assessed by the Impact of Event Scale-Revised in Chinese earthquake victims: Examining factor structure and its stability across sex. *Journal of Anxiety Disorder*, 25, 369-375.

World Health Organization, 2013. Health risk assessment from the nuclear accident after the 2011 Great East Japan earthquake and tsunami, based on a preliminary dose estimation. Geneva, Switzerland: WHO Press.

---

* This chapter is based on the following paper adding the latest data: Tsujiuchi, T., 2019. Post-traumatic Stress Due to Structural Violence after Fukushima Disaster. *Japan Forum*: doi:10.108 0/09555803.2018.1552308.

3   Mental Health / Public Health / Social well-being

Social Capital and Mental Health in a Major Disaster

Results of surveys and support after the Fukushima Daiichi nuclear power plant accident

Takahiro Iwagaki CSW, PSW, PhD [1][3] *(Social Medicine, Social Welfare),*
Takuya Tsujiuchi MD, PhD [2][3] *(Medical Anthropology),*
Atsushi Ogihara PhD [2][3] *(Social Medicine, Social Welfare)*

Key words: Social capital, mental health, Fukushima Daiichi nuclear power plant accident, social support

Abstract

Social capital is gaining attention for the role it can play in post-disaster reconstruction. The term "social capital" refers to concepts valued as parts of human relationships including trusting in others, high rates of cooperation, interpersonal networks, and participation in the community. Recent researches have reported that the risk of PTSD, depression and other mental disorders are low in regions rich in social capital when a disaster occurs.

This research project looked into the relationship between social capital and mental health as it pertains to evacuees escaping the Fukushima Daiichi nuclear power plant accident. Results showed that among both elderly subjects and mothers raising children, mental health was less likely to deteriorate the richer the subjects were in individual-level social capital.

It will be important for future disaster reconstruction policies to include the implementation of methods designed to foster social capital.

---

[1] Visiting Researcher, Advanced Research Center for Human Sciences, Waseda University
[2] Professor, Faculty of Human Sciences, Waseda University
[3] Waseda Institute of Medical Anthropology on Disaster Reconstruction (WIMA)

I. Introduction

Social capital is gaining attention for the role it can play in post-disaster reconstruction. In more familiar terms, social capital is an expression used to describe the connections people make with each other. The more general term "social overhead capital" refers to roads, dykes, and other infrastructure, while the more specific social capital means the capital that arises from human relationships, including having trust in others, high rates of cooperation, and interpersonal networks.

Aldrich (2015) researched the Great Hanshin-Awaji Earthquake (or Kobe earthquake) and while he reported no strong relationship between the speed of reconstruction and the scale of initial damage, he found that, in addition to population density and social and economic circumstances, participation in the community, high rates of cooperation, trust, and other forms of social capital did have a large effect. In other words, evacuations, cooperation and protection were went more smoothly for residents in areas rich in social capital, whereas these behaviors were not brisk in areas poor in social capital, and in such areas, it took more time to rebuild people's lives.

In addition, according to Tanaka, et al. (2010), incidents of "solitary death" occurred most frequently directly after people moved from temporary housing into homes reconstructed after the disaster. There were cases of low-independence elderly evacuees and others with financial difficulties continuing to live in evacuation centers and temporary housing until these facilities were shut down, and that group living had allowed resident's associations and volunteer groups to offer them protection, someone to speak to, group gatherings, and various other means of support. How-

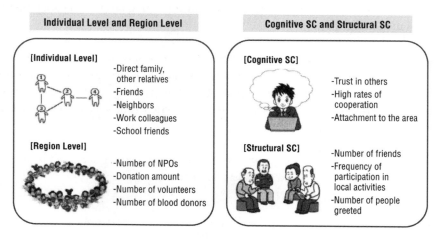

Figure 1. Types of social capital

ever, it is pointed out that the close community relationship that had been built was lost after people began moving individually into private residences, temporary housing, and rebuilt homes, suggesting that the danger of isolation would increase drastically. It is for this reason that it is important to build relationships with neighbors and friends even during the reconstruction period.

II. Social capital: definitions and types

The definition of social capital differs by academic field. American political scientist Robert D. Putnam (1993) defines social capital as the trust, norms, networks and other characteristics of social organizations that improve social efficiency by inducing cooperative behavior among individuals. The World Bank (2006) defines it as the systems, relationships, and norms that determine the quantity and quality of social connections. The Organization for Economic Co-operation and Development (OECD) (2001) defines it as networks of shared norms and values comprised up individuals with a shared understanding that contribute to the promotion of intra- and inter-group cooperation. Economist Yoji Inaba (2008) defines it as the trust, norms, and networks which have a mental externality. This vagueness in the definition of social capital has been described as one of its weaknesses (Inaba, Y., et al., 2014). However, it seems important that the concept is one that connects state of mind with social behavior.

Social capital is also classified into different types, the first of which defines it as either individual-level or region-level social capital (Fig.1). Individual-level social capital is made up of relationships focused on individuals, including those with family, friends, and neighbors. In contrast, region-level social capital is an evaluation of the levels of trust and cohesion among residents of a specific regional unit.

Individual-level social capital can be further classified into cognitive and structural types (Fig.1) Cognitive social capital is those behaviors that occur on a cognitive level, including trust in others, high rates of cooperation, attachment to the community/area, etc. Structural social capital is that capital which can be assigned an actual numerical value and viewed objectively, including number of friends, the frequency with which individuals participate in community activities, etc.

III. Disasters and social capital

Various research is being conducted world-wide on the importance of social capital during disasters, and much of it has proven that social capital has a powerful relationship with resilience in disaster areas (Aldrich, D.P., 2015). One particularly famous piece of research dealt with flooding in Morpeth, England in 2008 (Wind,

148   Part II - 3

T.R., Komproe, I.H., 2012). Researchers interviewed 232 survivors. They reported that the higher an area was in individual-level cognitive social capital, the lower the risk of post-traumatic stress disorder (PTSD), depression, and other anxiety disorders. Beaudoin (2007) studied the effects of Hurricane Katrina in the USA and reported that the more active a resident's social interaction at the individual level around the time of the disaster, the lower the risk of depression. In addition, Beiser, et al. (2010) surveyed survivors of violence in Nigeria and reported that the lower the level of individual social capital, the higher the rate of PTSD was found.

These results show us that residents continue to actively engage in mutual aid even after disasters occur in regions with extremely high levels of trust, cooperation, and community attachment, and that this behavior is thought to potentially minimize the incidence of secondary post-disaster damage.

IV. Relationship between social capital and mental health after the Fukushima Daiichi nuclear power plant accident

The authors conducted two surveys on the relationship between social capital and mental health of Fukushima evacuees who moved to the metropolitan Tokyo area. The surveys were conducted with individuals, so this report discusses the individual-level cognitive and structural social capital.

1. Survey of elderly individuals (Iwagaki, T., et al., 2017a)

The authors collaborated with the Shinsai Shien Network Saitama (SSN) in 2014 to conduct a survey of 3,599 households from Fukushima living in Saitama and Tokyo using self-administered questionnaires. A total of 772 responses were received (a response rate of 21.5%), and 229 responses corresponding to elderly individuals between 65 and 85 years of age were selected for analysis. The subjects were mainly from designated evacuation areas.

The Stress Response Scale 18 (SRS-18) was used to measure levels of mental health. The SRS-18 designates the threshold for an individual in a state of high-stress to be 32 points for men and 33 points for women (Suzuki, S., et al., 1997). Responses were sought for three questions: "Do you trust your neighbors?", "Will you be able to cooperate with your neighbors the next time a disaster occurs?" and "Do you feel pride in and attachment to the place you currently live?" Cognitive indicators for individual-level social capital were measured on a five-point scale: "completely agree," "somewhat agree," "cannot say," "somewhat disagree," "completely disagree." For structural indicators, subjects were asked to divulge how often they engage in hobbies, entertainment, sports and other community activities using one of

Social Capital and Mental Health in a Major Disaster 149

six levels: "two or three times a week," "once a week," "two or three times a month," "once a month," "a few times a year," and "never have participated." Subjects were asked how many of their neighbors they greet using one of four levels: "ten or more people," "five to nine people," "one to four people," and "no one." They were also asked whether they had participated in gatherings held for evacuees by answering either "yes" or "no."

Elderly individuals were targeted by this research because there are indications that drastic changes in lifestyle can easily cause health issues among the elderly, and that decreases in physical activity can result in a reduction of physical functionality and deterioration in mental health. Many of those evacuated from the designated exclusion zones have still not returned home by 2016, five years after the disaster. Radioactive waste material can be found in black flexible bulk containers stacked around their hometowns, and hospitals, supermarkets, and other parts of the infrastructure of life have yet to be restored. Neighbors are also unable to return. Houses have lain vacant for years, and many have suffered damage from termites, burglary, or wild animals, making the homes unsuitable for habitation.

We evaluated the stress of evacuees in this situation and found that 42% of men and 43% of women were in a "state of high stress."

Moreover, we used a multi-logistic model to analyze the relationship between high stress and each item related to social capital and calculated the odds ratio and 95% confidence interval. Social capital was analyzed at the individual level in terms of separate cognitive and structural indicators. Data was adjusted for sex, age, economic situations, the number of moves, and the existence of health issues before the disaster.

Table 1. Relationship between a high-stress group and cognitive social capital

Trust in Neighbors	Odds Ratio	95% Confidence Interval
High	1	
Medium	2.05	(1.00–4.20)
Low	5.19	(1.04–25.87)

Adjusted for age, sex, economic situations, the existence of health issues, and the number of moves

Table 2. Relationship between a high-stress group and structural social capital

Participation in Community event	Odds Ratio	95% Confidence Interval
2–3 times/week	1	
1 time/week–few times/year	2.70	(0.90–8.07)
Never participated	3.32	(1.06–9.15)

Adjusted for age, sex, economic situations, the existence of health issues, and the number of moves

150   Part II - 3

Table 3. Relationship between a depressed group and cognitive social capital

Trust in Neighbors	Odds Ratio	95% Confidence Interval
Can trust	1	
Cannot trust	1.85	(1.10–3.13)

Adjusted for age, academic history, economic situations, exercise habits, and concerns towards radioactive contamination.

As can be seen in Table 1, it is clear that respondents who answered "cannot trust neighbors" to the question regarding whether or not they can trust their neighbors (a form of cognitive social capital) were 5.19 times more likely to be at risk of high stress than respondents who answered that they "trust neighbors very much."

In addition, Table 2 clearly shows respondents who answered that they "have never participated" in community activities (a form of structural social capital) were 3.32 times more likely to be at risk of high stress than respondents who answered that they "participate in community activities two to three times a week."

2. Survey of mothers raising children (Iwagaki, T., et al., 2017b)

In 2015, in collaboration with NHK Sendai, the authors conducted a survey of 16,686 households in eight municipalities in Fukushima Prefecture using a self-administered questionnaire. A total of 2,862 responses were received (a response rate of 17.2%), and responses corresponding to 241 mothers under voluntary evacuation and currently raising children were selected for analysis.

The Center for Epidemiologic Studies Depression Scale (CES-D) was used to measure levels of mental health. The cut-off score for the CES-D is 16 points, with any score equal to or over 16 showing a trend towards depression. However, in surveys of Japanese subjects, 16 points has been indicated as being too low of a cut-off value, so a cut-off of 26 points was used as it has been determined to provide a more accurate evaluation of depression (Iwata, N., 2004). Social capital was analyzed in the same way analysis was conducted on the elderly subjects.

The reason for selecting subjects who had voluntarily evacuated was because there were indications that there was a higher risk of social isolation among mothers raising children who evacuated to locations outside the prefecture to protect their children from the effects of radiation (Yamane, S., 2013; Negayama, K., 2014; Toda, N., 2016). Family members differed in their perception of the risks of radiation exposure and the necessity of evacuating outside of the prefecture, which resulted in cases in which fathers stayed behind while mothers evacuated with their children. This increased the child-rearing burden on the mothers, and there were concerns about the deleterious effect of that on their mental health. Additional issues with securing

Social Capital and Mental Health in a Major Disaster   151

housing, financial burdens, and living in an unfamiliar area piled up, which indicated the possibility that mothers would become socially isolated.

Our research found a trend towards depression among 32.7% of the mothers surveyed. In addition, the data clearly showed that mothers who had evacuated only with their children were 2.41 times more likely to be at risk for depression than mothers who evacuated with their husbands, parents, or other family members.

Moreover, we used a multi-logistic model to analyze the relationship between high stress and each item related to social capital and calculated the odds ratio and 95% confidence interval. As in the survey of elderly individuals, social capital was analyzed at the individual level in terms of separate cognitive and structural indicators. Data was adjusted for age, academic history, marital status, household income, subjective feelings about health, and the existence of concerns about radiation exposure.

As shown in Table 3, it is clear that mothers who responded that they "cannot trust their neighbors" to the question regarding whether or not they can trust their neighbors (a form of cognitive social capital) were 1.85 times more likely to be at risk of suffering from depression than respondents who answered that they "can trust their neighbors."

In addition, Table 4 clearly shows that in terms of participating in community activities such as local mother's clubs and school PTA (a form of structural social capital), mothers who answered that they "do not participate" were 2.43 times more likely to be at risk of suffering depression than mothers who answered that they "do participate."

Table 4. Relationship between a depressed group and structural social capital

Participation in Community event	Odds Ratio	95% Confidence Interval
Do participate	1	
Do not participate	2.43	(1.02–5.78)

Adjusted for age, academic history, economic situations, exercise habits, and concerns towards radioactive contamination.

V. Discussion

The authors have demonstrated the effects of various psychological, social, and financial factors on PTSD, depression, and other mental health issues among evacuees and other victims of the Fukushima Daiichi nuclear power plant accident (Tsujiuchi, T., et al., 2012a; 2012b; 2016a; 2016b; Masuda, K., et al., 2013; Tsujiuchi, T.,

2012; 2014; 2015; 2016; 2017; Yamaguchi, M., et al., 2016). In this paper, we introduced two studies on individuals who evacuated to other prefectures from Fukushima after the nuclear accident (Iwagaki, T., et al., 2017a; 2017b), and both studies made clear that the existence of trusting relationships and community participation had a strong influence on mental health in the evacuation areas.

Koyama, et al. (2014) conducted a survey in Iwanuma city, Miyagi prefecture of evacuees from the Great East Japan Earthquake and reported that residents who received more counselling from other local residents and other social support had better mental health. Ohashi, et al. (2015) also showed through a post-disaster survey conducted in Rikuzentakata city, Iwate prefecture that evacuees with many social relationships had improved their mental state to some extent, and the existence of friends and other people with whom subjects could interact daily played a role in reducing great feelings of unhappiness. In this way, social capital is fostered by promoting participation in the community and increasing levels of trust among individuals through various methods of social support. Resident's associations, group meetings, volunteers, senior's clubs and various other community resources are available to the elderly, and it is necessary to put them in contact with such resources. It is also thought important to foster social capital by focusing on protecting those individuals who are at risk of becoming isolated.

As of 2016, there are reconstruction assistants in place in municipalities affected by the nuclear accident mainly conducting door-to-door visits and activities to bring people together. However, the scope of support required is wide-ranging, and it is difficult to respond to everything with only reconstruction assistants. Therefore, it is important to fortify the support and protection offered through collaborations between reconstruction assistants, municipalities and social workers both in evacuation destinations and areas where people have migrated, and public institutions such as government bodies and social welfare councils.

There is also support available for mothers who continue to raise their children in areas they evacuated to. Primarily, it is considered extremely important to help mothers obtain free time for themselves, so municipalities are offering short term child care, inexpensive transportation to day care facilities, domestic help, and other social services. The authors work with the Shinsai Shien Network Saitama (SSN), which holds social gatherings aimed at elderly disaster victims in addition to cooperating with the running of gatherings for mothers and children who have evacuated. As there is now childcare space available, visitors can now take their time in receiving living counselling and exchanging information. It is still necessary for healthcare providers and other supporters to become actively connected with such public social services and private support organizations.

Social capital was a key concept underpinning the practical societal care and support offered to evacuees from the nuclear accident and other victims of the great disaster, and it is expected that the concept will be able to be applied in the future in an increasingly super-aging or low-birthrate society.

VI. Conclusion

In order to improve mental health, it will be necessary for psychosomatic medical researchers to ask how to increase trust in neighbors and awareness of the necessity of mutual cooperation among people who have evacuated or migrated after a disaster. It is thought important to cooperate with public health nurses, social workers, local government officials, and policy makers to include the fostering of social capital as a part of disaster reconstruction planning, and to actively engage in social care and support through such means as increasing the number of neighbors one greets and promoting participation in shared hobbies, entertainment and other community activities.

References

Aldrich, D.P., 2014. Building Resilience: Social Capital in Post-Disaster Recovery. Ishida, Y., Fujisawa, Y., (Trans.), 2015. *Saigai fukkō ni okeru sōsharu kyapitaru to wa nanika.*, Minerva Shobō.

Beaudoin, C.E., 2007. News, social capital and health in the context of Katrina. *Journal of Health Care for the Poor and Underserved*, 18, 418-430.

Beiser, M., Wima, O., Adebajo, S., 2010. Human-initiated disaster, social disorganization and post-traumatic stress disorder above Nigeria's oil basins. *Social Science & Medicine*, 71, 221-227.

Inaba, Y., 2008. *sōsharu kyapitaru no senzai ryoku.* [The Latent Power of Social Capital.], Nihon Hyōronsha.

Inaba, Y., Omori, T., Kanamitsu, J., et al., 2014. *sōsharu kyapitaru "kizuna" no kagaku towa nanika.* [Social Capital: The Science of Interpersonal Ties.], Minerva Shobō.

Iwagaki, T., Tsujiuchi, T., Komaki, K., et al., 2017a. Relationships between Individual-level Social Capital Familial Relationships, and Mental Health in Mothers who have remained Voluntarily Evacuees Due to the Fukushima Nuclear Power Plant Accident. *Bulletin of Social Medicine*, 34, 21-29.

Iwagaki, T., Tsujiuchi, T., Masuda, K., et al., 2017b. Relationship between Individual Social Capital and Mental Health in Elderly who Left the Prefecture Due to the Fukushima Nuclear Power Plant Disaster. *Japanese Journal of Psychosomatic Medicine*, 57, 173-184.

Iwata, N., 2004. *CES-D Yokuutsu shakudo no shinri sokutei hō teki tokusei – kokusai hikaku no ōkina shōheki.* [Psychometric methodological characteristics of the CES-D depression scale: Major barriers to international comparisons.], Case Study meetings in the Japan Association for Research on Testing.

Koyama, S., Aida, J., Kawachi, I., 2014. Social Support Improves Mental Health among the Victims Relocated to Temporary Housing following the Great East Japan Earthquake and Tsunami. *Tohoku Journal of Experimental Medicine*, 234, 241-247.

Masuda, K., Tsujiuchi, T., Yamaguchi, M., et al., 2013. *Genshiryoku hatsudensho jiko ni yoru kengai hinan ni tomonau kinrin kankei no kihaku ka – Saitama ken ni okeru genpatsu hinansha daikibo ankēto chōsa wo motoni.* [Weakening social ties among neighbors following evacuation outside Fukushima Prefecture due to the nuclear power plant accident – Based on large-scale questionnaire survey of nuclear evacuees in Saitama Prefecture.], *Journal of Health and Welfare Statistics*, 60, 9-16.

Negayama, K., Hirata, S., Ishijima, K., et al., 2014. *Shinsai chokugo no hinan ni tomonau kazoku to kodomo no shinri.* [Psychology of families and children following post-disater evacuation.], Kamata, K., (Supervisor), Waseda University Earthquake Reconstruction Studies Editorial Committee (Ed.), *Shinsai go ni kangaeru – Higashi nihon daishinsai go to mukiau 92 no bunseki to teigen.* [Thinking after a disaster – 92 analyses and recommendations after the Great East Japan Earthquake.], Waseda University Press, pp. 311-322.

OECD, 2001. The Well-being of Nations: The Role of Human and Social Capital. Available from: http://www.oecd.org/site/worldforum/33703702.pdf [Accessed 9 Sep 2016]

Ohashi, K., Kondo, N., 2015. *Rikuzen Takata-shi ni okeru higashi nihon daishinsai kara no fukkō mirai zu.* [Future roadmap for reconstruction in Rikuzentakata after the Great East Japan Earthquake.], *The Japanese Journal for Public Health Nurse*, 71, 150-156.

Putnam, R.D., 1993. Making Democracy Work – Civic Traditions in Modern Italy. Princeton University Press. Kawata, J., (Trans.), 2001. *Tetsugaku suru Minshu Shugi – Dentō to Kaikaku no shimin teki kōzō.* [Philosophizing Democracy – Civil Structure of Tradition and Reform.], NTT Publishing.

Suzuki, S., Shimada, H., Miura, M., et al., 1997. *Atarashī shinri teki sutoresu shakudo (SRS18) no kaihatsu to shinraisei, datōsei no kentō.* [Development of a new stress response scale (SRS-18): A review of reliability and validity.], *Japanese Journal of Behavioral Medicine*, 4, 22-29.

Tanaka, M., Takahashi, C., Ueno, Y., 2010. *Ōkyū kasetsu jūtaku ni okeru "kodokushi" no hassei jittai to sono haikei.* [Actual incidents of "solitary death" in emergency temporary housing and a background: cases from the Great Hanshin-Awaji Earthquake.], *Journal of Architecture and Planning*, 75, 1815-1823.

The World Bank Annual Report, 2006. Available from: http://siteresources.worldbank.org/INTANNREP2K6/Resources/2838485-1158333614345/AR06_final_LO_RES.pdf [Accessed 9 Sep 2016]

Toda, N. (Ed.), 2016. *Fukushima genpatsu jiko, hyōryū suru jishu hinan sha tachi – jittai chōsa kara mita kadai to shakai teki shien no arikata.* [The Fukushima nuclear power plant accident. Voluntary evacuees adrift – Issues and social support methods from actual survey results.], Akashi Shoten.

Tsujiuchi, T., 2012. *Genpastu jiko hinansha no fukai seishin teki kutsū – kinkyū ni motome rareru shakai teki kea.* [Deep psychological distress of nuclear accident evacuees – Urgently required social care.], *Sekai*, 835, 51-60.

Tsujiuchi, T., Masuda, K., Chida, Y., et al., 2012a. Establishment of public-private cooperative system to support evacuees from the nuclear contaminated area: A case in Saitama Prefecture. *Japanese Journal of Psychosomatic Internal Medicine*, 16, 261-268.

Tsujiuchi, T., Yamaguchi, M., Masuda, K., et al., 2012b. *Genpatsu jiko hinansha no shinri, shakai teki kenkō – Saitama ken ni okeru chōsa kara.* [Psychological and social health of nuclear accident evacuees - From a survey conducted in Saitama prefecture.], *Depression Frontier*, 10, 21-31.

Tsujiuchi, T., 2014. *Shinkoku sa tsuzuku genpatsu jiko hisaisha no seishin teki kutsū; kikan wo meguru kunō to sutoresu.* [The deepening psychological trauma of nuclear accident victims: anxiety and stress about returning home.], *Sekai*, 852, 103-114.

Tsujiuchi, T., 2015. *Genpatsu jiko kōiki hinansha no torauma ni taisuru shakai teki kea no kōchiku.* [Constructing a system of social care to treat trauma for nuclear accident evacuees over a wide area.], *Japanese Journal of Molecular Psychiatry*, 15, 238-241.

Tsujiuchi, T., 2016. *Genpatsu jiko ga motarashita seishinteki higai – kōzō teki bōryoku ni yoru shakai teki gyakutai.* [Psychological trauma from the nuclear accident – Social abuse due to structural violence.], *Kagaku*, 86, 246-251.

Tsujiuchi, T., Yamaguchi, M., Masuda, K., et al., 2016a. High prevalence of post-traumatic stress symptoms in relation to social factors in affected population one year after the Fukushima nuclear disaster. *PLoS One*, 11: e0151807. doi: 10.1371/journal.pone.0151807.

Tsujiuchi, T., Komaki, K., Iwagaki, T., et al., 2016b. High-level Post-traumatic Stress Symptoms of the Residents in Fukushima Temporary Housing: Bio-psycho-social Impacts by Nuclear Power Plant Disaster. *Japanese Journal of Psychosomatic Medicine*, 56, 723-736.

Tsujiuchi, T., 2017. *Genpatsu saigai ga hisai jūmin ni motarashita seishin teki eikyō.* [Mental impact on residents affected by the nuclear disaster.], *Trends in the Sciences*, 22, 8-13.

Wind, T.R., Komproe, I.H., 2012. The mechanisms that associate community social capital with post-disaster mental health: A multilevel model. *Social Science & Medicine*, 75, 1715-1720.

Yamaguchi, M., Tsujiuchi, T., Masuda, K., et al., 2016. Social Factors Affecting Psychological Stress of the Evacuees Out of Fukushima Prefecture by the Cause of Nuclear Accident after the Great East Japan Earthquake – Suggestions from Longitudinal Questionnaire Survey. *Japanese Journal of Psychosomatic Medicine*, 56, 819-832.

Yamane, S., 2013. *Genpatsu jiko ni yoru "boshi-hinan" mondai to sono shien – Yamagata ken ni okeru hinansha chōsa no dēta kara.* [Issues with "mother-child evacuation" after the nuclear accident and support – From data gathered from surveys of evacuees in Yamagata Prefecture.], *Yamagata University Faculty of Literature and Social Sciences Annual Report*, 10, 37-51.

---

* This chapter is based on the following paper: Iwagaki, T., Tsujiuchi, T., Ogihara, A., 2017. Social Capital and Mental Health in a Major Disaster: Findings and Suggestions from the Survey and Social-support after Fukushima Nuclear Disaster. *Japanese Journal of Psychosomatic Medicine*, 57, 1013-1019.

4 | Mental Health / Community Health / Social Well-being

Weakening Social Ties among Fukushima Evacuees and Providing Support

Kazutaka Masuda CSW, PhD [1] [2] *(Studies of Social Work)*

Key words: social ties, neighborhood, post-traumatic stress disorder (PTSD), the impact of event scale-revised (IES-R)

I. Introduction

Three years have passed since the Great East Japan Earthquake (or Tohoku Earthquake) struck on 11 March 2011, and the people in the affected areas continue to rebuild. However, there are still many who are forced to live the life of evacuees long-term due to the effects of the disaster and the nuclear accident in Fukushima at the Tokyo Electric Power Company Nuclear Power Plant. The disaster caused widespread damage, and in addition, the accident at the Fukushima Daiichi Nuclear Plant resulted in the spread of radioactive material, and subsequent evacuation of many residents who left the prefecture to escape its effects. Those escaping the prefecture were separated from their local connections and community organizations and forced to make lives in new areas. This has led to concerns about people becoming isolated in the communities they have evacuated to – something that became a large issue after the Great Hanshin-Awaji Earthquake of 1995 (also known as the Kobe Earthquake). There is data showing a sharp increase in suicides in the period two to three years after the Kobe earthquake (Nishio, 2009), and researchers have been studying precautionary measures to take in relation to issues connected to isolation.

In a similar way, after the Tohoku Earthquake, there is a need for an effective support network to deal with the decrease in quality of life due to the evacuation and loss of community, and the degradation of mental health. Evacuees living in prefectures a long distance from their hometowns face greater difficulties in regard to loss of com-

---

[1] Lecturer, Department of Psychology and Social Welfare, School of Letters, Mukogawa Women's University
[2] Visiting Researcher, Waseda Institute of Medical Anthropology on Disaster Reconstruction (WIMA)

158   Part II - 4

munity and deteriorated relationships with neighbors when compared to those who evacuated within the prefecture, and the risk of isolation is estimated to be high. For that reason, we aimed to use surveys and data analysis to get a better understanding of the current mental health situation surrounding those individuals forced to evacuate to areas outside the prefecture after the Tohoku Earthquake, and to get a better grasp on how individuals are building relationships in the areas they evacuated to (an issue thought to have a knock-on effect on people's lives.) Our hope is that this work will allow us to provide recommendations for future support initiatives aimed at dealing with the societal isolation of disaster evacuees.

II. Research Methods

1. Outline and goals of the questionnaire survey

The Earthquakes and Human Sciences practical research team at Waseda University's Faculty of Human Sciences is led by Takuya Tsujiuchi. The team collaborated with a private support organization called the Saitama Earthquake Support Network (SSN) represented by Tadashi Inomata, and worked in cooperation with the Victim Support Division at Fukushima Prefecture's Living Environment Department to distribute a self-administered questionnaire in municipal information packages to households that evacuated from Fukushima to Saitama and Tokyo. The questionnaire was designed to get up-to-date understanding of the conditions of those who had evacuated from Fukushima due to either damage caused by the earthquake/ tsunami or the nuclear accident evacuees. This would be accomplished by getting a grasp of the extent of damage evacuees to Saitama and Tokyo suffered, and an understanding of their mental state. The aim was to encourage government bodies and other support organizations to provide more appropriate support (Tsujiuchi, et al., 2012). This paper uses a portion of the data gathered in that questionnaire to clarify the state of mental health among those evacuees and summarize the trends in social ties.

The survey was conducted between March and April 2014, and targeted 3,599 households in the survey area (with 772 responses received for a response rate of 21.5%), many of whom were forced to evacuate due to the nuclear power plant accident. In addition, Saitama and Tokyo were selected as the target of the survey for a few reasons: conditions in evacuation destinations outside of Fukushima Prefecture (Fukushima Prefecture, 2014), the fact that support had been continually offered in Saitama and Tokyo by the Earthquakes and Human Sciences practical research team at Waseda University's Faculty of Human Sciences, and the continued cooperation of the Fukushima Prefecture Disaster Countermeasure HQ support team for evacuees outside of the prefecture (headed by Saitama) making distribution of the questionnaires possible.

2. Survey items

The questionnaire was comprised of the following items that asked about: age; sex; address before earthquake; extent of damage to home; presence of tsunami damage; loss of employment due to earthquake; emergence of new illnesses after earthquake; necessity of nursing care for respondent and/or family; degree of post-traumatic stress symptoms; and number of relationships with neighbors before and after the disaster.

Awareness of post-traumatic stress disorder (PTSD) arose after the Kobe earthquake, and the Impact of Event Scale-Revised (IES-R) was used to determine the extent of post-traumatic stress symptoms. PTSD is seen as a stress disorder caused by trauma experienced during war, other conflicts, disasters, major accidents, crime, traffic accidents, etc., and it has been regarded as an important concept connected to mental health in past disasters in Japan and other countries. PTSD is defined using three characteristic types of symptoms: invasive symptoms (repeated/invasive painful memories of a traumatic event); avoidance symptoms (conscious and unconscious avoidance on the level of thoughts, emotions, and behaviors connected to a traumatic event); and hyperarousal symptoms (sleep disorders, irritability, anger, excessive caution and startle response). Each symptom type is thought to appear within one month of the occurrence of a traumatic event.

The IES-R used in this project is a measure frequently used in PTSD research since the 1980's, and it consists of 22 items in three subsections (with responses on a five-point scale). These items have been proven valid in different cultural contexts in its use as a standard through which stress conditions can be measured (Maercker and Schutzwohl, 1998; Asukai, et al., 2002). The version translated by Asukai (Asukai, 1999) was used here, and its reliability and validity had been verified. Higher scores in the IES-R correspond to higher levels of stress, and Asukai et al., suggested that a total score of 25 shows an increased risk of PTSD (Asukai, et al., 2002).

To determine the number of relationships with neighbors before and after the disaster, we used a question item measuring connections to neighbors from the National Survey of Lifestyle Preferences conducted by the Cabinet Office (Cabinet Office 2007). Specifically, regarding the depth of relationships with neighborhood residents, items were designated in descending order from close to distant, starting from "people you cooperate with, discussing each other's problems, lending everyday items, etc." to "people you speak with regularly on the street" and "people you greet or have minimal contact with." Respondents were asked to answer how many neighbors would fit in each classification for the periods "before the earthquake" and "after the earthquake."

3. Ethical considerations

Ethical considerations were addressed by enclosing with the questionnaire paper a request letter that explained that there was no requirement to fill out the questionnaire for those who did not consent to taking part, and that there would be no penalties for not taking part. In analyzing the data, respondent anonymity was protected by using coded questionnaires, and both the survey and analysis methods were approved by Waseda University's Ethics Review Committee on Human Research (Approval Number 2012-011.) In addition, data was handled with full consideration given to protecting privacy and was carefully stored to ensure no third party could gain access.

III. Results

1. Basic attributes of questionnaire respondents

Sex distribution of respondents was 385 male and 361 female. Many respondents were in the 50 to 79 age range, with the average age of respondents was 60.6 years old. For pre-disaster living location, the most common answer was Namie at 174, followed by Minamisoma at 130, and Futaba at 108. The majority of respondents evacuated from designated evacuation zones (with a total of 510 respondents having done so.) In addition, 7.3% responded that their homes were "completely destroyed", 14.6% answered "half-destroyed", 46.2% answered "partially destroyed", 22.3% answered that their homes suffered "no damage," and 6.6% responded "do not know." A total of 8.0% of respondents answered that their residences had been damaged by the tsunami to some extent. A total of 54.3% answered that they had experienced job loss caused by the disaster, and 43.3% answered that they were suffering from new illnesses that had appeared after the disaster. The survey also clarified that 14.6% of respondents had found it necessary to obtain nursing care either for themselves or for a member of their family.

2. IES-R scores

The average IES-R score of respondents in this survey was extremely high at 31.88 ± 21.5. In addition, 59.0% of respondents scored higher than 25 points, indicating that more than half of respondents were in a state of high stress and potentially suffering from PTSD.

3. Number of relationships with neighbors before and after the disaster

Survey data on number of relationships with neighbors before and after the disaster is displayed in Table 1 alongside the national averages. Pre-disaster numbers for "people you cooperate with, discussing each other's problems, lending everyday items, etc." show that 15.2% of respondents classified 10 or more neighbors within that group, much higher than the national average of 1.5%. A similar trend was seen

Weakening Social Ties among Fukushima Evacuees and Providing Support   161

for pre-disaster numbers for "people you speak with regularly on the street" and "people you greet or have minimal contact with," with a comparatively high percentage answering "10 or more".

Looking at the current post-disaster relationships with neighbors, 2.0% of respondents answered "10 or more" for "people you cooperate with, discussing each other's problems, lending everyday items, etc.," which is closer to the national average of 1.5%. The proportion who answered "0 people" was 60.2%, also closer to the national average of 65.7%. Including the ratios of respondents who answered "1 to 4 people" and "5 to 9 people," we see an overall trend towards the national average for post-disaster numbers. For the item "people you speak with regularly on the street," 35.3% answered "0 people," 52.3% answered "1 to 4 people", both of which are higher than the national average. Additionally, for the item "people you greet or have minimal contact with," 15.7% answered "0 people," and 56.9% answered "1 to 4 people," for a total of 72.6% of responses.

Table 1. Results: pre-disaster and post-disaster relationships with neighbors, alongside data from National Survey of Lifestyle Preferences (2007) (Units: %)

Depth of neighbor relationship		Pre-disaster	Post-disaster	National Average (# responses in brackets)
People you cooperate with in everyday life	0 people	16.7%	60.2	65.7 (2,211)
	1 - 4 people	50.9%	34.0	28.0 (942)
	5 - 9 people	17.1%	3.8	4.8 (162)
	10 people	15.2%	2.0	1.5 (51)
People you speak with regularly on the street	0 people	8.3%	35.3	33.3 (1,119)
	1 - 4 people	42.3%	52.3	33.4 (1,122)
	5 - 9 people	24.4%	8.1	19.2 (644)
	10 people	25.0%	4.3	14.1 (474)
People you greet or have minimal contact with	0 people	3.5%	15.7	13.1 (439)
	1 - 4 people	28.3%	56.9	25.7 (861)
	5 - 9 people	21.6%	17.9	25.6 (857)
	10 people	46.6%	9.4	35.6 (1,193)

Note: National Average data tabulated specially from National Survey of Lifestyle Preferences (2007) conducted by Cabinet Office.

4. Mental effect of weakened social ties

We used the results of this survey to determine what sort of psychological burden was placed on evacuees through the breakdown of their communities due to the evacuation, particularly on those who experienced an extreme drop in the number of close neighbors who they described as being "people you cooperate with in everyday life" Respondents who answered "10 or more" for that category before the disaster but answered "0 people" for current post-disaster relationships were categorized as

162   Part II - 4

the "Weakened Social Ties" group. All other respondents were placed in a second group named "Other," and the difference in mean IES-R scores for each group (ttest) was calculated. The analysis covered 47 individuals in the Weakened Social Ties group and 618 individuals in the Other group, and unanswered items were excluded. The results showed an average total score of 44.6 for those in the Weakened Social Ties group, and an average of 30.1 in the Other group. The difference in means was calculated and a statistically significant difference was confirmed at 0.1% (t(663) = 4.12, p < 0.001).

5. Individual attribute factors that affected the weakening of ties with neighbors who respondents "cooperate with in everyday life"

The analysis showed that individuals who saw an extreme weakening in social ties saw a corresponding increase in stress. Binomial logistic regression analysis was conducted to determine individual attributes that may have served as factors in increasing the possibility of weakened social ties. For the analysis, the dependent variable was set at 1 for the Weakened Social Ties group and 0 for the Other group. Forward selection (likelihood ratio) analysis was conducted on these independent variables: age; sex (female=0, male=1); extent of damage to home (none/partial=0, half/complete=1); presence of tsunami damage (none=0, some=1); loss of employment due to earthquake (no loss=0, loss=1); emergence of new illnesses after earthquake (no=0, yes=1); necessity of nursing care for respondent and/or family (no= 0, yes=1); degree of post-traumatic stress symptoms; and number of relationships with neighbors before and after the disaster. Results showed that sex (p<0.01, odds ratio (OR) = 3.95), existence of tsunami damage (p<0.01, OR = 3.93), loss of employment (p<0.05, odds ratio (OR) = 2.88), emergence of illness (p<0.05, OR = 3.41), and requirements for nursing care (p<0.05, odds ratio (OR) = 2.50) were factors that influenced the weakening of social ties.

IV. Discussion

1. Mental health of evacuees living outside Fukushima three years after the disaster as determined from IES-R scores

The high IES-R scores recorded during this survey three years after the disaster clearly show that the long-term evacuation due to the earthquake, tsunami, and nuclear accident continues to have an enormous psychological effect on evacuees. Comparing to past disasters in Japan, the average resident IES-R score 13 months after the Niigata Chuetsu earthquake was 14.3 ± 14.8, with 20.8% of respondents having a score over 25 points (Naoi, 2009). In addition, three years and eight months after the Kobe earthquake, a survey conducted among those living in temporary and rebuilt houses found the average resident's IES-R score to be 22.5 ± 16.8, with 39.5% scoring over 25 points (Kato et al., 2000). It is necessary to consider the time the measurements were taken and social conditions, so the numbers obtained in previous studies cannot be simply compared to the numbers determined in this research, but what can be said is that these results are extremely high (Yamazaki et al., 2009; Tanno et al., 2011). IES-R scores show levels of stress and the potential that an individual is experience PTSD, but that does not mean that high scores result directly in a diagnosis of PTSD; the existence of PTSD must be left to the judgement of a specialist medical professional. At the very least, this research clearly shows that evacuees living outside the prefecture are living in a state of high stress three years after the disaster.

The reasons for the high IES-R scores of evacuees living outside of the prefecture include the direct damage caused by the earthquake, and the fact that they are being forced to live outside the prefecture with no clear futures. For these evacuees, the disaster is not something that happened in the past – it is a state that continues, and that can be inferred from the high IES-R scores obtained during this survey. Therefore, there will be strong demand for continued support into the future to ameliorate the psychological suffering and monitor stress levels among evacuees.

2. Relationship between mental health and weakened social ties

This research showed that more than 15% of evacuees were unable to secure relationships based on even the most minimal of interactions, i.e. "the greeting level," with neighbors in the areas to which they evacuated, and there are strong concerns about individuals in those regions becoming isolated. This clearly illustrates the breakdown of community ties built before the earthquake and shines a light on the living conditions of evacuees as they deal with weaker social ties than they had previously. Some evacuees have been subject to bullying and harassment for simply being evacuees, and it could be said that people's caution regarding their evacuee status has prevented them from building new social ties in the communities in which they now live. In addition, it is still unclear whether or not they will be able to return to Fukushima, or how long they will have to live in their new communities, and that uncertain future is expected to have had an effect on their ability to create relationships in the communities they evacuated to. Naturally, the distance people place between themselves and the local community varies, and such individuality must be respected. However, after considering the trends in suicide rates and isolation problems after the Kobe earthquake, and considering how people will continue to live in their new communities, we must take seriously the fact that more than 15% of people responded that they have no one around them with whom they can exchange even the most minimal of greetings, and we must think about future means of providing support.

In addition, more than 80% of respondents answered that before the earthquake, they had at least one neighbor with whom they could discuss their problem, lend and borrow everyday items, and generally support each other in their lives, but more than half of those respondents now respond that they have zero neighbors with whom they have such a close relationship. These facts show us that people have been forced to undergo large changes in how they live compared to before the disaster, when their neighbors played a large social support role in their lives. It is thought that the sense of loss connected to the breakdown of that neighborly social support network is stronger when people are unable to adapt flexibly to such changes. Currently, the numbers corresponding to "people you cooperate with in everyday life" is trending towards the national average, which can be interpreted as meaning that the closeness of relationships being built in these new communities is reaching the maximum possible, but for the evacuees, the pre-disaster/post-disaster relationship gap is large, and that may have a large influence on their mental health. Indeed, in order to determine the psychological influence of weakening of social ties, we compared IES-R scores for the Weakening Social Ties group (for whom the number of close neighborly relationships dropped drastically) and the Other group, and total IES-R scores were significantly higher among those in the Weakened Social Ties group.

3. Individual attributes that affected the weakening of ties with neighbors who people "cooperate with in everyday life"

The analysis showed that sex, existence of tsunami damage, loss of employment, emergence of illness, and requirements for nursing care were all attributes that suggested a high possibility for weakened social ties. In more specific terms, the potential risk for experiencing a weakening in social ties was: 3.95 times higher for men than women; 3.93 times higher for those who suffered tsunami damage; 2.88 times higher for those who lost jobs; 3.41 times higher for those who discovered new illnesses post-disaster, and 2.50 times higher for those who had to receive nursing care for themselves or a family member.

Previous research has looked into social relationships for elderly males, and it indicated that many aspects depend on long-term relationships cultivated after meeting at a workplace or school (Koyano, 2000). Our survey showed something similar. The average respondent age was 60 years old, and after the evacuation caused a physical separation from others with whom respondents had enjoyed long relationships, some evacuees found it difficult to build relationships in their new communities. The increased risk among individuals who suffered the effects of the tsunami is assumed to have arisen from people who had built close relationships in coastal areas with neighbors in the fishing and other industries. After the disaster, they lost that common ground and ended up suffering weakened social ties because of it. Continuing on, regarding the items on loss of employment, appearance of new illnesses, and necessity of nursing care, it is thought that these experiences would have led to motivational and behavioral issues that would make building new relationships more difficult and thereby lead to weakened social ties.

4. Future methods of support

The results of this research suggest that living support is an urgent issue that must take into account the mental burden of evacuees living outside Fukushima having lost their communities and the weakened social ties in their new communities. With more than 15% of evacuees being unable to build relationships of even the minimal depth of "offering greetings," there are concerns about isolation in the communities evacuees have moved to. In addition, considering that many evacuees are living in a state of high stress, it seems necessary to quickly consider future means of intervention, which will also contribute to the prevention of suicide and solitary death. At that point, it will be important to be cautious in regard to resistance to the term "evacuee" and the stigma surround it, and to remain conscious of personal lifestyles and prevent excessive intervention that disregards individual circumstances. With these points in mind, opportunities for connecting with local communities can be created. In addition, relationships with neighbors cannot be built overnight. It takes time to build trust, so it seems necessary to construct a provisional monitoring system using certain public resources in order to provide distress-free and problem-free support. We believe it particularly necessary to proactively engage in outreach for evacuees with attributes corresponding to weaker social ties, and to conduct active investigations designed to gain a grasp of the current situation and provide timely intervention when needed.

Currently, local governments and private support organizations hold a variety of charity rebuilding events, consultation sessions, and gatherings for evacuees to come together, thereby helping to prevent isolation and provide a means for people to maintain the community connections they had before the disaster struck. However, there are issues disseminating information about these sorts of gatherings and events, and it has been pointed out that there are also issues with people physically getting access, which makes it difficult for some evacuees to attend these events due to their own individual circumstances. Over the three years since the disaster, the lives of evacuees have become more individual, with regional and personal differences arising that have led to the appearance of limitations in the intensive resource-driven support offered thus far. This is why it will be absolutely necessary for future support to include outreach functionality capable of responding to the individual needs of evacuees, and coordination of resources and information provision catered to the differing circumstances. Naturally, it is necessary to provide support tailored to individual needs and coordinated by professionals with the ability to adjust local resources and understand the conditions in which evacuees live, to address mental burdens caused by complex and individually-unique factors. However, there are limits to the what individual professions can keep watch over, so again, it is essential to have the support of local residents who can help ensure early detection of needs and risks and provide evacuees with someone nearby to speak to when they need it. That is simply another reason why there is a powerful demand for coordination based in the opinions of both evacuees and locals and a proactive support structure aimed at building new communities, in order to gain a better understanding of the distance between local residents and the evacuees who have joined them in their communities.

5. Limitations and issues

This research targeted evacuees who evacuated from Fukushima Prefecture to Saitama and Tokyo, so the results do not illustrate the situation faced by all evacuees. It has been suggested that there are numerous voluntary evacuees and others unknown to the Fukushima Prefecture Living Environment Department Victim Support Division, making it difficult to generalize these results. For this reason, it is necessary to engage in continued analysis based in these results and continue to research methods of resolving problems that arise.

Acknowledgments

I would like to express my gratitude to the organizations that cooperated in performing this study. In addition, I am deeply indebted to all of those who responded to the questionnaire despite the difficulties they continue to face.

This research was made possible by funding from the Welfare and Medical Service Agency's social welfare promotional subsidy project, the MEXT-Supported Program for the Strategic Research Foundation at Private Universities, and a project "returning the benefits of cerebral and psychological science back to society" run by the Waseda University Organization for University Research Initiatives (represented by Hiroaki Kumano).

Weakening Social Ties among Fukushima Evacuees and Providing Support 167

References

Asukai, N., 1999. *Fuan shōgai, gaishōto sutoresu shōgai (PTSD)*. [Anxiety Disorder, Post-Traumatic Stress Disorder (PTSD).], *Clinical Psychiatry Special Issue*, 28, 171-177.

Asukai, N., Kato, H., Kawamura N., et al., 2002. Reliability and validity of the Japanese-language version of the impact of event scale-revised (IES-R) - four studies of different traumatic events. J *Nerv Ment Dis*, 190, 175 - 182.

Cabinet Office, 2007. *Heisei 19 nen ban kokumin seikatsu hakusho (Tsunagari ga kizuku yutakana kokumin seikatsu)*. [2007 National Lifestyles White Paper (building a rich national lifestyle through connecting with each other).]

Fukushima Prefecture website, *Fukushima ken kara kengai e no hinan jyōkyō*. [Evacuation situation outside of Fukushima Prefecture.] Available from: http://www.pref.fukushima.lg.jp/uploaded/attachment/276444.pdf, [Accessed 10 July 2018]

Kato, H., Iwai, K., 2000. Posttraumatic stress disorder after the Great Hanshin-Awaji Earthquake: assessment by the structured interview to the survivors. *Medical Journal of Kobe University*, 60 (2), 27-35.

Koyano, W., Nishimura, M., Ando, T., Asakawa, T., Hotta, Y., 2000. *Toshi dansei kōreisha no shakai kankei*. [Social relationships among urban elderly males.], *Japanese Journal of Gerontology*, 22 (1), 83-88.

Maerker, A., Schutzwohl, M., 1998. Assessing mental effects of traumatic events: the impact event scale-revised. *Diagnostica*, 44, 130 - 141.

Naoi, K., 2009. Local Mental Health activity after the Niigata Chuetsu Earthquake – findings of investigations performed 3.5 months and 13 months after the earthquake, and analysis about the risk factor of PTSD, *Japanese Bulletin of Social Psychiatry*, 18, 52 - 62.

Nishio, A., Akazawa, K., Shibuya, F., et al., 2009. Influence on the suicide rate two years after a devastating disaster: A report from the 1995 Great Hanshin-Awaji Earthquake. *Psychiatry and Clinical Neurosciences*, 63(2), 247 - 250.

Tanno, H., Yamazaki, T., Matsui, Y., et al., 2011. *2007 nen Niigata ken chūetsu oki jishin no hisai kaigo shisetsu shokuin no sutoresu hannō*. [Stress response among disaster care facility staff after 2007 Niigata Chuetsu Offshore Earthquake.] *Japanese Journal of Disaster Medicine*, 16, 19-26.

Tsujiuchi, T., Yamaguchi, M., Masuda, K., et al., 2012. *Genpatsu jiko hinansha no shinri · shakai teki kenkō – Saitama ken ni okeru chōsa kara*. [Psychological and social health of nuclear accident evacuees - From a survey conducted in Saitama prefecture.], *Depression Frontier*, 10, 21-31.

Yamazaki, T., Tanno, H., 2009. *2004 nen Niigata ken chūetsu jishin no hisai kangoshi no sutoresu hannō – Niigata chūetsu jishin wo taiken shita kangoshoku no ankēto kekka kara*. [Stress response of nurses after the 2004 Niigata Chuetsu Earthquake – results of questionnaire on nurse practitioners active during Niigata Chuetsu earthquake.] *Japanese Journal of Disaster Medicine*, 14, 157 - 163.

*This paper was based on the following paper using the latest data: Kazutaka Masuda, Takuya Tsujiuchi, Maya Yamaguchi, Kanade Yamashita, Haruka Nagatomo, Shikiko Nagumo, Saki Awano, et al., 2013. *Genshiryoku hatsudensho jiko ni yoru kengai hinan ni tomonau kinrin kankei no kihakuka – Saitama ken ni okeru genpatsu hisansha daikibo ankēto chōsa wo motoni*. [Weakening social ties among neighbors following evacuation outside Fukushima Prefecture due to the nuclear power plant accident – Based on large-scale questionnaire survey of nuclear evacuees in Saitama Prefecture.], *Journal of Health and Welfare Statistics*, 60 (8), 9-16, Health, Labour and Welfare Statistics Association.

5   Mental Health / Community Health / Social Well-being

Relationships between psychological, social, and economic factors behind mental problems caused by experiencing disasters, and how to best provide social welfare support

Tsutomu Taga MA[1,2] *(Social & Clinical Psychology, Social Welfare)*

Key words: disaster victims, post-traumatic stress disorder (PTSD), depression, social workers, psychologists

I. Introduction

Between March and April 2012, Tsujiuchi (2016) conducted a mail-in post-traumatic stress disorder (PTSD) survey of 2,011 households that had evacuated from Fukushima Prefecture to Saitama Prefecture after the accident at Tokyo Electric Power Company's Fukushima Daiichi Nuclear Power Plant. The results of the survey showed that chronic physical and/or mental conditions, worries about maintaining a livelihood, loss of employment, and concerns about compensation were societal factors with a statistically significant effect on disaster victims suspected of suffering from PTSD. In addition, Tsujiuchi (2015) conducted a similar mail-in survey in February 2013 that found that the effect of economic difficulties, concerns about compensation, aggravation of chronic medical conditions, development of new medical conditions, and lack of support from neighbors were statistically-significant factors among 2,425 households affected by the disaster and living in temporary housing within Fukushima Prefecture. The previous studies suggest that there is a link between PTSD and socio-economic factors.

---

[1] Senior Researcher, Research Team for Promoting Independence of the Elderly, Tokyo Metropolitan Institute of Gerontology
[2] Visiting Researcher, Waseda Institute of Medical Anthropology on Disaster Reconstruction (WIMA)

Disaster victims suspected of suffering from PTSD are thought to be more vulnerable to stress, and thereby thought to require even more support when living as evacuees. However, there is a need for support framework aimed at evacuees vulnerable to stress even when they are not suspected of PTSD. In this paper, we will turn our attention to symptoms of depression as indicators of vulnerability to stress. First, we focus on the combination of suspected PTSD alongside symptoms of depression, and potential relationships between psychological, social, and economic factors. Second, we consider the hypothesis that there is a generational difference in the relationships to those factors. Age groups are herein defined as young (15-34 years old), middle-aged (35-64), and elderly (65 and over). It is thought that there are differences in what the three age groups worry about regarding psychological, social, and economic issues following disasters, and differences in levels of vulnerability.

In order to present a generalized analysis of PTSD and depression, this paper analyzes an integrated data set gathered from three survey sources: Fukushima Prefecture residents primarily affected by the man-made nuclear disaster at Tokyo Electric Power Company's Fukushima Daiichi Nuclear Power Plant (16,686 surveys distributed, 17.2% response rate); Iwate Prefecture residents affected by the natural disaster of the tsunami (12,187 surveys distributed, 21.1% response rate); and Miyagi Prefecture residents affected by the tsunami (27,271 surveys distributed, 20.6% response rate). These surveys were conducted between January and March 2015 through mail surveys sent to disaster victims living in and out of their home prefectures. The Impact of Event Scale-Revised (IES-R) was used to analyze PTSD factors, and the Center for Epidemiological Studies Depression Scale (CES-D) was used to analyze depression.

Before the analysis was begun, the differences in the average PTSD and depression scale scores were reviewed statistically for each of the three prefectures. No significant differences were found between the three prefectures on either scale, and regardless of disaster experienced, the suspected levels of PTSD and depression were the same for victims from all three prefectures (see Table 1). In addition, the correlation coefficient between the CES-D and IES-R scores was calculated, and as expected, a strong correlation between PTSD and depression was found ($r = .697, p = .000$). This suggests that symptoms of depression may be complicated by PTSD symptoms, which further suggests that it is appropriate to create a variable that combines both PTSD and depression.

Table 1. Comparing average IES-R and CES-D scale scores in three affected prefectures

	IES-R	CES-D
Iwate	0.40	0.55
Miyagi	0.39	0.57
Fukushima	0.41	0.56
Variance analysis	$F(2, 9557) = 0.916$	$F(2, 9118) = 1.711$
Significance test	n.s. (p = .400)	n.s. (p = .181)

*Average values were compared as some scale/score items were missing.

With the above in mind, this paper aims to discuss how social welfare support should be provided to victims whose PTSD symptoms complicate symptoms of depression and victims displaying symptoms of depression when not suspected of suffering from PTSD.

II. Analytical Method

1. Survey Subjects
Respondents residing in Iwate, Miyagi, and Fukushima prefectures at the time of the disaster were classified into three age groups: young (15-34 years old), middle-aged (35-64), and elderly (65 and over).

2. Creating Dependent Variables
The international standard IES-R was used as the PTSD scale. A binary variable was assigned by setting the cut-off score at 25 points, with a score 25 or higher corresponding to potential PTSD in a subject (Horowitz, 1979; Weiss, et al., 2004; Asukai, et al., 2002). The CES-D used in epidemiological surveys around the world was used as the depression scale. A binary variable was assigned in this case with a cut-off score of 16, and 16 points or more corresponding to potential depression in a subject (Radloff, 1977; Shima, et al., 1985). Using these two binary variables, survey subjects were classified into four groups defined by presence or absence of PTSD symptoms and presence or absence of depression symptoms: [No PTSD/No depression]; [No PTSD/ Suspected depression]; [Suspected PTSD/No depression]; and [Suspected PTSD/ Suspected depression].

3. Selecting independent variables
Multiple regression analysis was conducted with IES-R and CES-D scores as dependent variables, and independent variables were selected. Factor analysis was conducted on the survey items comprised of multiple questions, and where factor extraction was possible, the average value for each factor was used. Pre-selection independent variables can be found in Table 2.

Table 2. Independent variables (before selection)

Category	Main variables
Disaster conditions	Residence, tsunami/bereavement experience, length of time living in disaster area, etc.
Living conditions	Livelihood, income, debt, savings, etc.
Employment status	Occupation, industry, unemployment, experience working at nuclear power plant, etc.
Residential environment	Form of ownership, residence type, layout, floor space, intentions regarding residence, satisfaction with residential environment, etc.
Physical health	Condition, tobacco use, alcohol use, exercise, index of activity capacity for the elderly, educational history, chronic disease requiring treatment, etc.
Matters concerning radiation	Knowledge of exposure, worries, examinations, thoughts regarding restarting nuclear power plants, etc.
Family situation	Household size, household composition, marital status, nursing care, living apart, family relationships, etc.
Mental health	Psychological changes, mental health care, etc.
Status of co-habiting children 12 and under	Number of children/grandchildren, age, gender, family relationship, wake-up time, bedtime, Post Traumatic Stress Symptom for Children 15 items (PTSSC-15: Tominaga et al, 2001), parental bereavement, etc.
Conditions as living as evacuee	Information availability, means of dealing with distress, having a confidant, relationship with community, relationship with relatives, frequency of leaving the house, status of community activities, participation in evacuee exchange meetings, local character, etc.

Gender, age group (young, middle-aged, elderly), disaster area (Iwate, Miyagi, Fukushima) variables were set via forced entry, and variables considered to be connected to the dependent variables for each survey item were selected using the stepwise method. Finally, variables selected for each item were input simultaneously, and independent variables were selected.

4. Investigation of related psychological, social, and economic factors

In order to investigate the strength of the relationships between the combined PTSD/depression values and psychological, social, and economic factors, multiple logistic regression analysis was performed with the four PTSD/depression groups as dependent variables. The healthy group (No PTSD/No depression) was set as the reference variable, and the multiple logistic regression analysis was repeatedly performed for each age group.

III. Results

1. Simple Tabulation

A simple tabulation of the data for the three age groups (young, middle-aged, and elderly) can be found in Table 3.

Table 3. Simple tabulation

	Age Group (Note a)	# responses Young	# responses Middle-aged	# responses Elderly	Ratio Young	Ratio Middle-aged	Ratio Elderly	Statistical significance (Note b)	Significance test (Note c)
Suspicion of PTSD & Suspicion of depression	No PTSD/No depression	52	195	88	40.6%	31.5%	43.6%	0.004	**
	Suspected PTSD/No depression	11	43	19	8.6%	6.9%	9.4%		
	No PTSD/Suspected depression	21	152	28	16.4%	24.6%	13.9%		
	Suspected PTSD/Suspected depression	44	229	67	34.4%	37.0%	33.2%		
Gender	Male	32	290	136	25.0%	46.8%	67.3%	0.000	***
	Female	96	329	66	75.0%	53.2%	32.7%		
Disaster Area (Prefecture)	Iwate	20	104	42	15.6%	16.8%	20.8%	0.593	n.s.
	Miyagi	59	258	82	46.1%	41.7%	40.6%		
	Fukushima	49	257	78	38.3%	41.5%	38.6%		
Experienced tsunami	Yes	43	221	101	33.6%	35.7%	50.0%	0.001	**
	No	85	398	101	66.4%	64.3%	50.0%		
Worried about living expenses	Yes	113	506	135	88.3%	81.7%	66.8%	0.000	***
	No	15	113	67	11.7%	18.3%	33.2%		
Level of financial difficulty	Very worried	49	192	35	38.8%	31.0%	17.3%	0.000	***
	Somewhat worried	58	294	102	45.3%	47.5%	50.5%		
	Not worried	21	133	65	16.4%	21.5%	32.2%		
Existence of pre-disaster medical condition requiring treatment	Yes	31	171	144	24.2%	27.6%	71.3%	0.000	***
	No	97	448	58	75.8%	72.4%	28.7%		
Reason for ending/not accepting mental health care	Issue not very serious	66	260	101	51.6%	42.0%	50.0%	0.029	*
	(N/A)	62	359	101	48.4%	58.0%	50.0%		
	Treatment wouldn't resolve issues	27	220	45	21.1%	35.5%	22.3%	0.000	***
	(N/A)	101	399	157	78.9%	64.5%	77.7%		
	Don't know where to get help	19	59	20	14.8%	9.5%	9.9%	0.194	n.s.
	(N/A)	109	560	182	85.2%	90.5%	90.1%		
PTSSC-15	Child/grandchild PTSD score (average)	1.3	1.8	1.9	–	–	–	0.000	***
	Child/grandchild depression score (average)	1.2	1.6	1.8	–	–	–	0.000	***
Relationship with community in evacuation area	Lack of mutual trust (average)	3.0	2.9	2.7	–	–	–	0.000	***
	Sense of isolation (average)	1.3	1.8	1.9	–	–	–	0.000	***
Information necessary to living in evacuation area	Local government brochures	74	382	138	57.8%	61.7%	68.3%	0.118	n.s.
	(N/A)	54	237	64	42.2%	38.3%	31.7%		
Total		128	619	202	100.0%	100.0%	100.0%		

Note a: Age group definitions – Young: 15-34; Middle-aged: 35-64; Elderly: 65 and over

Note b: Variance analysis used to test differences in average values, otherwise Goodman & Kruskal's τ value was used.

Note c: *** = $p < .001$, ** = $p < .01$, * = $p < .05$, n.s. = no significance

174   Part II - 5

1) Dependent variables
The numbers of respondents with no suspected depression in spite of suspected PTSD were low across all age groups. The young and elderly age groups had the highest number of respondents with neither PTSD nor depression symptoms. The middle-aged group had a relatively large number of respondents with suspected depression, independent of the presence or absence of PTSD symptoms.

2) Independent variables
Female respondents outnumbered male respondents in the young age group by a statistically significant margin, while male respondents outnumbered female respondents in the elderly group. With the young and middle-aged groups, a large number of respondents did not experience the tsunami, while the ratio of those who did experience it to those who didn't was the same for the elderly group. Many respondents in the young and middle-aged groups are worried about maintaining their livelihoods and experience financial difficulties, while those numbers were low among the elderly group. A large number of elderly respondents had been receiving necessary treatment for a medical condition before the disaster, while the opposite was true for the young and middle-aged groups. A relatively large number of middle-aged respondents indicated that they had ended/not accepted mental health care despite the severity of the mental care problems they faced because "Treatment wouldn't resolve issues." Mental care issues were not as severe among young and elderly respondents, and a comparatively large number of respondents indicated their belief that receiving mental health care would aid in recovery.

2. Relationships between psychological, social, and economic factors with regards to the combined suspected PTSD/depression variable by age group
Table 4 presents the relationships between psychological, social, and economic factors with regards to suspected PTSD and suspected depression by age group.

1) Suspected PTSD/No depression group
Based on the healthy group (no PTSD/no depression), resident disaster area was the factor most likely to place young respondents in this group. With Fukushima respondents set at 1, Iwate respondents were 36.6 times, and Miyagi respondents 17.1 times more likely.

The factor most likely to place middle-aged respondents in this group was when respondents did not know where or from whom they could receive mental health care, with such respondents 4.0 times more likely to end up in this group.

For the elderly age group, respondents with pre-disaster medical conditions requiring treatment were 4.0 times more likely to end up in this group.

Table 4. Relationships between psychological, social, and economic factors with regards to suspected PTSD and suspected depression by age group

Dependent Variables (Note a)		Young (15-34)						Middle-aged (35-64)						Elderly (65 and over)					
Suspected PTSD →		Yes		No		Yes		Yes		No		Yes		Yes		No		Yes	
Suspected depression →		No		Yes		Yes		No		Yes		Yes		No		Yes		Yes	
Independent Variables		Sig. (b)	Exp (B)	Sig. (b)	Exp (B)	Sig. (b)	Exp (B)	Sig. (b)	Exp (B)	Sig. (b)	Exp (B)	Sig. (b)	Exp (B)	Sig. (b)	Exp (B)	Sig. (b)	Exp (B)	Sig. (b)	Exp (B)
Gender	Male	0.179	4.202	0.574	1.449	0.649	0.70	0.243	0.75	0.996	1.00	0.382	0.79	0.367	1.86	0.330	1.75	0.833	0.89
	Female																		
Disaster Area (Prefecture)	Iwate	*0.022*	35.57	0.684	0.65	0.257	3.58	0.799	0.91	0.540	0.69	*0.048*	0.42	0.503	0.48	0.867	0.87	0.117	0.23
	Miyagi	*0.042*	17.14	0.334	0.48	0.065	4.32	0.264	1.40	0.591	1.27	*0.007*	0.40	0.909	0.90	0.442	0.58	0.180	0.36
	Fukushima																		
Experienced tsunami	Yes	0.185	3.77	0.244	2.33	0.137	3.10	0.529	0.83	0.799	1.12	*0.015*	2.24	0.592	1.57	0.860	1.12	0.399	1.86
	No																		
Worried about living expenses	Yes	0.588	2.17	0.478	2.86	0.084	10.13	0.116	2.09	0.210	2.25	0.308	1.69	0.597	0.62	0.885	0.88	0.168	0.31
	No																		
Level of financial difficulty	Very worried	0.069	0.07	0.203	5.92	0.568	0.55	0.845	0.90	0.557	0.68	0.062	2.69	0.209	4.20	0.591	1.90	*0.018*	13.25
	Somewhat worried	0.059	0.07	0.224	4.97	0.493	0.51	0.617	1.25	0.233	0.49	0.977	1.01	0.906	0.90	0.936	1.08	0.236	2.87
	Not worried																		
Existence of predisaster medical condition requiring treatment	Yes	*0.039*	8.54	0.336	2.14	0.768	1.27	*0.049*	1.77	0.143	1.83	0.603	1.18	*0.045*	3.99	0.238	1.89	*0.001*	8.78
	No																		
Reason for ending/not accepting mental health care (Inverted)	Issue not very serious	*0.045*	0.13	0.508	0.60	*0.002*	0.10	0.681	1.12	0.512	0.77	*0.000*	0.20	0.824	1.16	0.981	1.01	*0.002*	0.18
	N/A																		
	Treatment wouldn't resolve issues	0.451	2.42	0.245	0.23	*0.010*	8.47	*0.000*	2.90	*0.009*	2.92	*0.002*	2.60	0.277	2.42	0.163	0.20	0.078	3.26
	N/A																		
	Don't know where to get help	0.280	3.62	0.344	2.27	0.547	1.75	0.325	1.64	*0.021*	4.02	0.485	1.46	0.769	1.51	0.311	3.03	0.444	2.21
	N/A																		
PTSSC-15	Child/grandchild PTSD score	0.395	1.96	0.602	0.76	0.413	1.56	*0.020*	1.62	*0.025*	1.97	*0.000*	3.07	*0.014*	4.02	0.187	1.88	0.057	2.41
	Child/grandchild depression score	0.667	0.63	0.276	2.05	0.097	3.04	0.739	1.08	0.768	0.91	0.482	0.84	0.696	0.78	0.205	1.96	0.088	2.40
Relationship with community in evacuation area	Lack of mutual trust	0.651	0.73	0.348	1.55	0.011	3.52	0.057	1.45	0.834	0.94	*0.000*	2.11	*0.028*	0.34	0.604	1.24	0.431	0.74
	Sense of isolation	0.975	1.02	0.060	1.96	0.516	1.23	*0.001*	1.64	0.250	1.28	*0.000*	1.78	0.253	1.40	*0.019*	1.93	*0.014*	1.95
Information necessary to living in evacuation area (Inverted)	Local government brochures	0.611	0.62	0.673	0.76	0.559	0.68	0.688	0.90	0.171	0.61	0.288	0.74	0.719	0.79	0.504	1.53	0.254	0.53
	N/A																		
Intercept		0.245	—	0.002	—	0.000	—	0.003	—	0.233	—	0.000	—	0.56	—	0.006	—	0.016	—
Nagelkerke (Pseudo R2)		0.647						0.519						0.609					
AIC (model goodness of fit)		304.584						1262.034						432.454					

Note a: Reference variable for dependent variables = No PTSD/No depression.
Note b: Statistical significance p < .05 shown by underline.

176   Part II - 5

2) No PTSD/Suspected depression group

Based on the healthy group (no PTSD/no depression), there were no statistically significant factors that increased likelihood of young respondents being placed in this group.

The factor most likely to place middle-aged respondents in this group (at 2.9 times) was when respondents ended/did not accept mental health care because "treatment wouldn't resolve issues."

The factor most likely to place elderly respondents in this group (at 1.9 times) was when they felt a sense of isolation from the community in their evacuation area.

3) Suspected PTSD/Suspected depression group

Based on the healthy group (no PTSD/no depression) the factor most likely to place young respondents in this group (at 9.8 times, 0.10 times inverted) was when they ended/did not accept mental health care despite the severity of the mental health issues they faced.

The factor most likely to place middle-aged respondents in this group (at 5.1 times, 0.20 times inverted) was when they ended/did not accept mental health care despite the severity of the mental health issues they faced.

The factor most likely to place elderly respondents in this group (at 13.3 times) was when respondents were "very worried" about financial difficulties.

IV. Discussion

1. Reviewing social welfare support measures for those suspected of PTSD/depression

This paper makes no mention of psychological support for those affected by PTSD/depression, but does discuss the possibility of providing support through social welfare services.

1) Suspected PTSD/No depression group

This group is made up of individuals with no depression coinciding with PTSD. As PTSD is a form of psychological trauma, social welfare support is not expected to be very effective in resolving it. For example, for individuals in the young age group, the most strongly related psychological/social/economic factor for this group was having experienced the disaster in Iwate or Miyagi prefectures. The percentage of affected homes that were completely destroyed stands at more than 90% in Iwate, approximately 70% in Miyagi, and approximately 10% in Fukushima. Witnessing the extent of the destruction due to collapse and flooding of their communities is thought to have been a factor in the emergence of PTSD. Additional factors were also strongly related to placement in this group, such as witnessing PTSD symptoms in children and having pre-existing medical conditions requiring treatment at the time of the disaster, neither of which can be very effectively handled through the provision of social welfare support.

2) No PTSD/Suspected depression group
Individuals in this group showed no symptoms of PTSD, but did present symptoms of depression. Looking at the psychological, social, and economic factors connected to this group we find that middle-aged and elderly respondents shared a sense of isolation from the communities to which they had evacuated. For middle-aged respondents, a distrust of mental health care effectiveness and presence of PTSD symptoms in children were also associated with membership in this group. Variables such as social gatherings for disaster victims and availability of professional counselling sessions were excluded through the process of variable selection using multiple regression analysis. There is demand among the victims for a new form of social welfare support.

While no statistically significant factors were found that placed young respondents in this group, there seems to be a strong relationship to financial problems. When looking for financial issues particular to the young age group, it was found that median savings for this group were on the order of 1,000,000 yen, while median savings for the middle-aged and elderly groups were on the order of 5,000,000 yen (Kruskal-Wallis test, $p = .000$). Average age of eldest child under 12 for the young age group was 5.4 years, while for the middle-aged group it was 8.2 years and the elderly group (in this case, grandchildren) it was 8.5 years (F (2, 1, 394) = 78.04, $p = .000$). It is thought that a low amount of savings was a particularly large source of stress for those raising children. However, it may be difficult to alleviate or eliminate such financial worries through the provision of social welfare support.

3) Suspected PTSD/Suspected depression group
This group has a comparatively larger number of related psychological, social, and financial factors. This is particularly true of the middle-aged group, for which more than half of the factors are connected. The most major characteristic of the middle-aged group is its strong relationship to the disaster in Fukushima. The man-made disaster at the Tokyo Electric Power Company's Fukushima Daiichi Nuclear Power Plant had an effect on PTSD at the time of the disaster, but there are also indications that there may have been an influence on the discovery of depression symptoms while these individuals were living as evacuees. Other factors included a distrust of mental health care and a lack of trust in the communities to which they evacuated,

and a sense of isolation from those communities. Attitudes towards mental health care and relationships with the communities in the evacuation areas tended to be shared by the young age group as well. The distrust of mental health care among respondents in the young and middle-aged groups may actually be a symptom of depression. Another reason for the distrust may lie in the limitations inherent to attempting to support mental health and living problems separately. It seems that it is necessary to aim to resolve mental health issues in the process of helping people deal with problems of everyday life.

Meanwhile, factors strongly connecting elderly respondents to this group included level of financial difficulty and the pre-existence of a medical condition requiring treatment at the time of the disaster. However, it may be difficult to provide social welfare support aimed at alleviating or eliminating financial worries or issues related to chronic medical conditions.

2. Combined psychological and social welfare support measures

The preceding section discusses the potential that lies in providing social welfare support, through a new means of support that combines livelihood support provided by social welfare with psychological support through mental health care. While psychological issues can generally be handled through mental health care, when psychological, social, and economic factors become interconnected, there is the potential to improve people's physical lives concurrently with improvements to mental health by integrating mental health care into social welfare. One example can be found in the case of providing support to young or middle-aged individuals who are isolated and distrust their local communities. In this case, psychologists can perform outreach activities (i.e. through home visits) in order to treat PTSD in children, but in addition to that, by collaborating with social workers with their welfare standpoint, an effort can be made to bring parents into the community through connecting their children to local resources and people. Mental health issues should not be treated only through psychological care. Instead, by incorporating social welfare support into such care, it becomes possible for both psychological and social welfare issues to be improved in an integrated fashion. This is particularly true as psychological issues in individuals and their families often tend to be hidden behind community social welfare issues. Currently in the planning stages are collaborations between social workers and medical professionals, and between psychologists and medical professionals, but the idea of collaboration between social workers and psychologists remains an issue to be discussed in the future.

References

Asukai, N., et. al., 2002. Reliability and validity of the Japanese-language version of the Impact of Event Scale-Revised (IES-R-J): Four studies on different traumatic events. *The Journal of Nervous and Mental Disease*, 190, 175-182.

Horowitz, M., et al., 1979. Impact of Event Scale: A Measure of Subjective Stress. *Psychosomatic Medicine*, 41(3), 209-218.

Radloff, L.S., 1977. The CES-D scale: A self-report depression scale for research in the general population. *Applied Psychological Measurement*, 1(3), 385-401.

Shima, S., et al., 1985. *Atarashī yokuutsu sei jiko hyōka syakudo ni tsuite*. [A new self-report depression scale.], *Psychiatry*, 27(6), 717-723.

Tsujiuchi, T., 2015. Mental health impact of the Fukushima Nuclear Disaster: Post-traumatic stress and psycho-socio-economic factors. United Nations University Fukushima Global Communication Programme Working Paper Series:1-7. Available from: http://i.unu.edu/.../ias.unu.ed.../news/12850/FGC-WP-8-FINAL.pdf

Tsujiuchi, T., et al., 2016. High prevalence of post-traumatic stress symptoms in relation to social factors in affected population one year after the Fukushima Nuclear Disaster. *PLoS One*, 11(3), e0151807. doi:10.1371/journal.pone.0151807.

Weiss, D.S., 2004. The Impact of Event Scale-Revised. In: Wilson, J.P., Keane T.M. (Eds.), Assessing psychological trauma and PTSD (Second Edition). The Guilford Press, New York: pp168-189.

6 Mental Health / Family Health / Community Health

Psychology of Families and Children Evacuated after Disaster

Koichi Negayama PhD[*1][*6] *(Developmental Human Ethology),*
Shuzo Hirata MA[*2] *(Developmental Psychology, Child Welfare),*
Konomi Ishijima MA[*3][*6] *(Developmental psychology),*
Ryuhei Mochida MA[*4] *(Developmental psychology),*
Yuko Shiraishi MA[*5] *(Developmental psychology)*

Key words: evacuation, family, children, parent, stress, moving

I. Goals and Methods of the *Kasasagi* Project Survey

1. Aims

The term "disaster" covers natural disasters such as earthquakes and typhoons, and man-made disasters such as war and acts of terror, and they cause people to experience major stress. In recent years, some research has been conducted into developmental issues faced thereafter by people who have experienced such disasters (Cherry, 2009; Masten and Narayan, 2011; Masten and Osofsky, 2010). The Tohoku disaster was a complex combination of the 2011 off the Pacific coast of Tohoku earthquake, tsunami, and subsequent nuclear power plant accident. It was a disaster of unprecedented scale that severed ties within families and communities, and there is great value in considering the developmental impact the disaster had on individuals who experienced it.

Since the immediate aftermath of the 2011 Tohoku Earthquake, Koichi Negayama has led the Human Developmental Ethology Laboratory at Waseda University's Faculty of Human Sciences in its research of families who moved to the Kanto area just after

---

[*1] Professor, Faculty of Human Sciences, Waseda University
[*2] Lecturer, Department of Child Studies, Sendai Seiyo Gakuin College
[*3] Research Associate, Department of Education for Childcare, Tokyo Kasei University
[*4] Visiting Researcher, Advanced Research Center for Human Sciences, Waseda University
[*5] Research Fellow, Center for Brain Science, Institute of Physical and Chemical Research (RIKEN)
[*6] Waseda Institute of Medical Anthropology on Disaster Reconstruction (WIMA)

their homes were damaged in the earthquake or tsunami, or due to the nuclear power plant accident. The *Kasasagi* Project was launched with the goal of working with the families to find solutions to the various psychological and behavioral problems that arose. While the project is small-scale, it has engaged in various means of support after families were forced away from the environments and communities they knew, and even forced to live apart.

One aspect essential to the continued activity of this post-disaster project was the fact that Negayama was both a victim of, and a receiver of support after, the 1995 Kobe earthquake. Negayama (2010) described how a survey was conducted immediately after the Kobe earthquake into parent-child relationships at the moment of the disaster. It clarified that essential aspects of parent-child relationships are manifested by earthquake phenomena. The present study expanded that perspective by extracting the fundamental aspects within families and between parents and children, as well as clarifying the relationship between child-rearing and communities, insofar as they relate to the Tohoku earthquake and subsequent evacuations. It was hoped that this could potentially lead to better support for evacuee families.

The *Kasasagi* Project continues to engage in activities to help parents and children better adapt through questionnaires and interviews conducted with evacuee families, behavioral observation of children, making of puppet plays by children of evacuee families and children already living in the communities, and other methods. Among them, this paper utilizes the results of a questionnaire conducted slightly less than one year after the disaster among families who had evacuated to Saitama to clarify the situation faced by the families with small children, issues of adaptation they have and other points, and to review means of providing them with support.

2. Methods

Questionnaire items: family situation at time of disaster, time/reason for evacuation, changes in family situation after evacuation, time/reason for subsequent moves, feelings regarding people remaining in Tohoku, predictions for the future, methods/frequency of contact with separated family members, current worries, etc.

Collaborators: Due to privacy concerns regarding protection of personal information, it was difficult to gain direct access to information on families that evacuated, so the team explained the purpose of the research to the evacuee response departments at each municipality in Saitama Prefecture, and requested that they act as intermediaries. Later, 945 questionnaires and return envelopes were delivered to the municipalities that granted permission, and starting roughly eight months after the disaster, the questionnaires were distributed to evacuee families in each area by their local municipalities between November 2011 and January 2012, resulting in a total of 248 anonymous responses (26.2% response rate). This survey was conducted after receiving the approval of the Waseda University Academic Research Ethical Review Committee.

II. Survey Results

1. Evacuation conditions

Respondents to the questionnaire described above were between 21 and 91 years old, with an average age of 52.38 (SD 18.16). This age distribution can be found in Figure 1, which shows that the largest group of respondents was in their 30s, followed by another peak of respondents in their 50s. Men made up 38% of respondents and women 60% (the remainder was unspecified). In terms of position in the household, 46.5% specified "householder," 35.9% specified "spouse of householder," 9.4% specified "child of householder", and 3.3% specified "parent of householder."

This survey was conducted by municipalities within Saitama Prefecture so the vast majority of respondents were naturally residents of Saitama Prefecture, but some respondents were residents of other prefectures. Table 1 shows a breakdown of only those respondents who specified that they were either householders or spouses of householders. Furthermore, among such respondents, it also shows the number and percentage of respondents from whom those respondents who did not specify their place of residence are excluded. Looking at the living conditions of respondents at the time of the survey, 64 of 70 householders (91.4%) responded that they were living in Saitama, while of householder spouses who responded, all 76 responded that they were living in Saitama. Among householder respondents, a high percentage (86.4%) answered that their spouses were also living in Saitama. However, a peculiarity arose in the answers of householder spouse respondents living in Saitama, among whom 36 or approximately half (49.3%) of the 73 responses stated that the householder was living in Fukushima Prefecture. In other words, the families that evacuated to Saitama Prefecture could be categorized into two general groups: families in which both husband and wife evacuated together, and families in which the householder remained in Fukushima while the spouse evacuated.

Table 2 shows the changes in family composition before and after the evacuation among families that moved to Saitama due to the disaster. A brief glance shows that a number of spouses no longer live together, and there is also similar trend visible in regard to children and grandchildren, particularly among householder respondents. Additionally, the data indicates another trend particularly among householder spouses for having stopped living with their parents-in-law and started living with their own parents. This shows us that the earthquake disaster and nuclear power plant accident caused major changes in family composition, particularly between married couples and between parents and children.

At the time of the survey, 90 families – approximately one third of the evacuated families – had moved four or more times, and moreover, the median time of their fourth move was April, the month after the disaster. This illustrates just how many families were forced to move repeatedly and hastily in a short period of time.

As previously mentioned, respondents covered a broad range of ages between 21 and 91 years old. Although all have been described as "evacuee families," the differences in age makes it difficult to describe them as a uniform group. Therefore, in regard to their initial moves, we categorized the families by how their living situation changed, and split them into sub-groups defined by sex and age. The living situation groups were: "still living together," "from living apart to living together," "from living together to living apart," and "still living apart/absent" (Fig. 2). This illustrates how the disaster served as a catalyst for many families to decide to start living apart. Among male respondents, a peak is seen among those in their 50s and 60s who ended up living apart, whereas among women, that peak is conspicuous among respondents in their 30s. These peaks correspond to the peaks seen in the age distribution shown in Fig. 1, and it can be inferred that these respondents had some reason for breaking up their families during the evacuation.

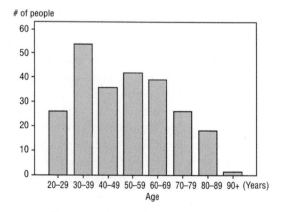

Figure 1. Age distribution of respondents

Psychology of Families and Children Evacuated after Disaster   185

Table 1. Residence of respondent and spouse (at time of survey)

Place of Residence	Householder provided response		Householder spouse provided response	
	Householder address	Householder spouse address	Householder address	Householder spouse address
Saitama	64 (91.4)	38 (86.4)	27 (37.0)	76 (100.0)
Fukushima	2 (2.9)	2 (4.5)	36 (49.3)	0 (0.0)
Miyagi	2 (2.9)	0 (0.0)	1 (1.4)	0 (0.0)
Ibaraki	1 (1.4)	0 (0.0)	1 (1.4)	0 (0.0)
Yamanashi	1 (1.4)	1 (2.3)	0 (0.0)	0 (0.0)
Niigata	0 (0.0)	1 (2.3)	2 (2.7)	0 (0.0)
Tochigi	0 (0.0)	1 (2.3)	1 (1.4)	0 (0.0)
Okayama	0 (0.0)	0 (0.0)	1 (1.4)	0 (0.0)
Yamagata	0 (0.0)	0 (0.0)	1 (1.4)	0 (0.0)
Chiba	0 (0.0)	0 (0.0)	1 (1.4)	0 (0.0)
Tokyo	0 (0.0)	0 (0.0)	1 (1.4)	0 (0.0)
Hyogo	0 (0.0)	0 (0.0)	1 (1.4)	0 (0.0)
Nagasaki	0 (0.0)	1 (2.3)	0 (0.0)	0 (0.0)
Total	70 (100.0)	44 (100.0)	73 (100.0)	76 (100.0)

(Note: Percentages shown in parentheses.)

Table 2. Changes in family composition among families living in Saitama from before the evacuation to ten months after

Position in home at time of disaster	Changes from pre-evacuation until ten months after	Family Member					
		Own parent	Spouse Parent	Spouse	Minor child	Adult child	Grandchild
Householder	No change	94	99	78	93	82	90
	Start living together	1	2	0	4	2	1
	Stop living together	8	3	26	6	19	12
	Total	103	104	104	103	103	103
Householder spouse	No change	74	70	31	79	78	85
	Start living together	8	4	1	3	1	1
	Stop living together	5	14	55	6	8	1
	Total	87	88	87	88	87	87
Householder child	No change	7	22	21	20	19	21
	Start living together	1	0	0	0	1	1
	Stop living together	15	1	1	2	3	1
	Total	23	23	22	22	23	23
Householder parent	No change	9	10	9	9	7	8
	Start living together	0	0	0	1	1	1
	Stop living together	1	0	1	0	2	1
	Total	10	10	10	10	10	10
Other	No change	8	6	7	10	8	7
	Start living together	2	0	0	0	0	0
	Stop living together	0	4	3	0	2	3
	Total	10	10	10	10	10	10

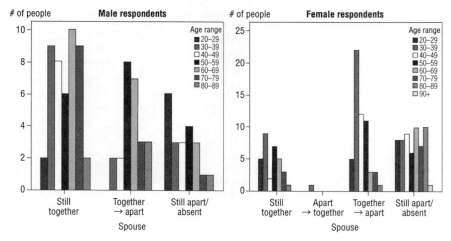

Figure 2. Changes in living situation decided upon by evacuee families at time of first move

2. The evacuation process

There was a drastic drop in responses for individuals who had moved five times or more, so the data on those who had moved up to four times was subject to more detailed analysis. First, there is the question of what location was selected as a destination, but a majority of families selected an evacuation center as their first location to which they would evacuate (Table 3). Additional responses included "automobile," which many selected for their first move, perhaps doing so only with the clothes they had on them. Some families moved temporarily to their homes in Fukushima. This is perhaps less that people were daring to live in the affected areas, and more that there were many cases of families temporarily gathering together at those locations. It became gradually more common for people to rely on different acquaintances and borrow/rent space from them, but by the 4th move, there were still a certain number of people choosing to stay at evacuation centers.

Table 4 shows how people's reasons for moving changed over time depending on the number of moves made. The percentage shown is the ratio of responses detailing the specific reasons for each residential move. According to these responses, half of evacuee families were forced to evacuate, either due to external instruction or voluntarily, in order to escape from the nuclear power plant accident and the damage caused by radiation released during that accident. The damage wreaked by the earthquake and tsunami was immense, but the additional severity of the impact of the nuclear power plant accident can be seen in these facts and in the unusual numbers on Fukushima Prefecture found in Table 1.

Additional responses included, particularly at the beginning, worries about tsunamis and aftershocks, the destruction of homes, and difficulties in maintaining basic living conditions due to cold temperatures or supply issues, which suggests that relocation was necessary in order to survive. Worries about radioactivity remained a large factor behind moving, but gradually the response "evacuation destination found" began to increase in frequency, alongside another more ambivalent trend, an increase in the frequency of the response "difficult to remain." We see how families moved into the homes of relatives and acquaintances with only the clothes on their backs, and eventually began seeking more stable places to live and moved out. Table 3 shows an increase in the trend of people looking for a place to support themselves, perhaps a choice that arose from the desire for a location that would offer a higher quality of life, and from the ambivalence of feeling that it was "difficult to remain" where they were.

Fig. 3 shows how, when asked about their hopes for future places of residence, respondent answers tended to fall into two broad categories – "I want to return to Tohoku" and "I don't know" – thereby illustrating the dilemma the families face. Needless to say, those who responded with "I don't know" were reserving judgement as no evaluation could be made regarding the future of the nuclear power plant or the effects of the radioactivity. This too shows the difficult futures faced by evacuee families. In contrast, less than 10% of respondents answered positively that they "want to remain in their current location," suggesting that the situations the evacuee families have found themselves in are unstable and harsh.

The evacuee families in Kanto also have a variety of feelings about the people still left in Tohoku. Figure 4 summarizes those feelings and presents one trend that can be seen as positive, with responses including "They are trying hard," "I miss them," and "I want to help." However, there were also responses in which respondents chose items which included negative elements, including "I feel sorry for them," "I feel bad for leaving," and "They should evacuate." Here too we find a kind of ambivalence.

Table 3. Change in destination

	1st move	2nd move	3rd move	4th move
Valid responses	246	227	184	135
Destination (in %)				
Evacuation center	52	26.9	14.7	12.6
Automobile	10.2	1.8	1.1	0
Hotel/ryokan	1.6	6.2	4.9	5.9
Home of parent/grandparent/great-grandparent	6.1	5.3	5.4	1.5
Home of son/daughter	4.9	7.5	12.0	10.4
Home of other relative/acquaintance	12.6	29.1	29.3	25.2
Own home	0	1.8	6.0	12.6
Home in Fukushima	6.1	3.1	1.1	0
Other	6.5	18.5	25.5	31.9
Total	100	100	100	100

Table 4. Change in reasons for moving

	1st move	2nd move	3rd move	4th move
Valid responses	185	151	112	70
Reason (in %)				
Restricted area, instructions to escape indoors, instructions from municipality	23.2	9.3	0.9	0
Nuclear accident, fleeing from/worries of radioactivity	27.6	20.5	12.5	7.1
Home completely destroyed	1.6	0.7	0	0
Aftershocks	1.1	0.7	0	0
Tsunamis	2.2	0	0	0
Cold, supplies, gasoline (basic living crisis)	4.3	1.3	2.7	5.7
Protect family (have infant children)	0.5	1.3	2.7	0
Evacuation destination found (relatives/acquaintances/evacuation centers)	6.5	9.9	12.5	12.9
Evacuation destination found (independent residence)	2.7	7.3	16.1	24.3
Work/study	4.3	9.3	13.4	7.1
Live with family	1.6	3.3	0	5.7
Worries about physical/mental health	5.4	4	6.3	1.4
Difficult to remain	8.1	14.6	15.2	24.3
Evacuation center closed, forced eviction from hotel after end of cost-free period, etc.	1.1	1.3	2.7	2.9
Nowhere to live/go	0.5	4	2.7	1.4
Costly	0.5	0.7	0.9	0
Other	8.6	11.9	11.6	7.1
Total	100	100	100	100

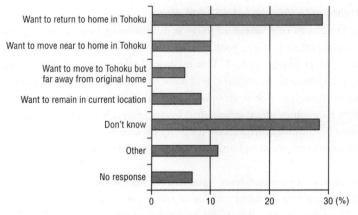

Figure 3. Hopes for the future

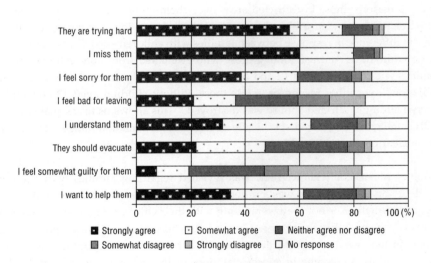

Figure 4. Feelings about people remaining in Tohoku

3. Cohabitating with children aged 12 and under

The central theme of our *Kasasagi* Project is determining how to provide support to families – specifically families with young children – dealing with the earthquake and nuclear power plant accident. This includes looking into what effect the experiences of the disaster and evacuation will have on child development, what problems are unique to families with such small children, and what sort of support can be offered from a developmental ethological perspective. During this research, we tried to find answers to those questions by focusing on families with children aged 12 and under and comparing them to families without such children.

Fig. 5 shows how responses were categorized into whether families had lived in restricted or non-restricted areas and the results show how the reasons for evacuation differed depending on whether or not a family had children aged 12 and under. The figure shows us that the reasons for evacuation were completely different between those living in what became restricted areas and those in non-restricted areas. For obvious reasons, those in restricted areas overwhelmingly selected "lived in designated or recommended evacuation area" as their reason for evacuating, and there was no difference in response between families with children aged 12 and under and those without. In contrast, among those who evacuated from non-restricted areas, families with children aged 12 and under overwhelmingly selected "worries about radiation" over other responses, while those without children aged 12 and under overwhelmingly selected "house was destroyed." This allows us to say that families with small children reacted specifically strongly to the radiation dangers caused by the nuclear power plant accident.

Another remarkable characteristic was revealed regarding families with children aged 12 and under – there was a difference found between fathers and mothers in regard to whether or not they were living with their children. Fig. 6 shows respondents who were either living or not living with children aged 12 and under by age group in ten-year increments, depending on whether or not couples were living together or apart (keeping in mind separations including death, divorce, etc.) What becomes immediately clear is that when the male partner in a couple was living elsewhere, the numbers of children aged 12 and under living with them was low across all age groups. On the other hand, for couples living together, not a few men in their 30s and 40s were cohabiting with children aged 12 and under. Similarly, in the case of female partners living elsewhere, relatively high numbers of women in their 30s were cohabiting with children aged 12 and under. Elderly respondents can be assumed to be grandparents and not parents.

On the other hand, when it comes to women, things are totally different. Many women were cohabiting with children aged 12 and under whether or not they were living with their partners. A remarkable peak can be observed among respondents in their 30s, and there is an overwhelmingly large number of cases of women, i.e. mothers, who evacuated to Saitama without their partners but with children aged 12 and under. This tells us eloquently how, when choosing to evacuate, a remarkable number of mothers chose to flee in order to protect their children from the dangers of radiation.

Finally, regarding people's feelings on those remaining in Tohoku, some significant differences were found between those living with children aged 12 and under and those not. Even more interesting is that there were also differences in trends in those significant differences based on whether or not a respondent was living in Saitama with their spouse or not (Table 5).

There was a stronger trend towards answering "They are trying hard" among those living as couples with children aged 12 and under, compared to those without. For those living separately, there was a stronger tendency for those with children aged 12 and under to respond, "I feel bad for leaving," "They should evacuate" or "I feel somewhat guilty for them." In other words, for respondents living with children, a conflicting trend was found, with those living with spouses having stronger positive feelings about people in Tohoku and those living without spouses having stronger negative feelings. As previously mentioned, for families with small children and particularly mothers in their 30s living in non-restricted areas, it can be inferred that there were numerous cases of mothers voluntarily evacuating with their children while fathers remained behind to work. In those cases, evacuees living elsewhere seem to have felt as if they had inexcusably left their families and neighbors behind. Such families may face unique hardships and have special worries, so careful consideration is required when providing them with support.

Finally, we asked respondents to provide written statements regarding any problems or worries they had at the time of the questionnaire, and we touch upon that here. We were able to classify the statements into seven categories: radiation/earthquakes; poor physical/mental health; life in the places to which they evacuated (at home/ school); living conditions, meals etc. in the disaster area; financial issues; emotional distance between direct family and other relatives; and future prospects. We specifically look at those applied to the respondents themselves, their children, spouse, parents/grandparents, and grandchildren.

Regarding the respondents themselves, many had difficulties or were worried about financial issues, poor physical/mental health, life in the places to which they evacuated, and future prospects. However, only two provided responses that corresponded to emotional distance between direct family and relatives, suggesting that those evacuees were more concerned with things directly linked to their lives and survival than they are about interpersonal relationships. Regarding children, the largest number of responses (33) were regarding life in the places to which they evacuated, followed by radiation/earthquakes. These respondents were worried about fitting in to their new schools and communities, and about possible injury due to radiation. Regarding spouses, the largest number of responses fell under the category of poor physical/mental health. Female respondents seemed to be thinking about their spouses' lives in the disaster areas, and the proportion of the respondents who answered that they were particularly worried about what their spouses were eating and about potential emotional distance between family members and other relatives was comparatively higher than the females giving other responses. Many respondents were worried about the physical and mental health of parents and grandparents, and while there were few responses mentioning grandchildren, there was a comparatively high number of worry about the lives of their grandchildren in the places to which they had evacuated.

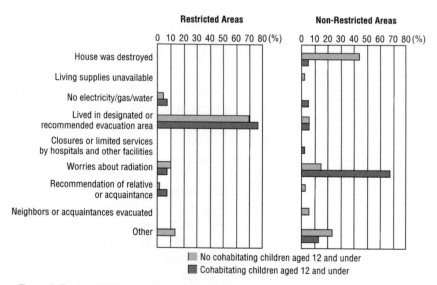

Figure 5. Regional differences in correspondence between presence of small children and reason for evacuation

Psychology of Families and Children Evacuated after Disaster   193

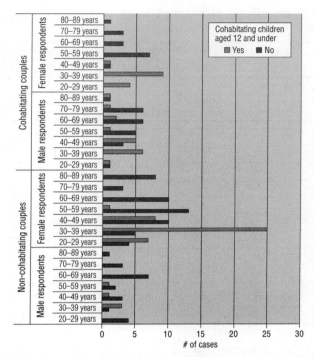

Figure 6. Correspondence between cohabitation/no cohabitation with spouse and children aged 12 and under

194   Part II - 6

Table 5. Differences in feelings towards those left in Tohoku as dependent on presence of children aged 12 and under

	Saitama respondents living with spouses						Saitama respondents not living with spouses					
	Freq.	Mean	SD	DoF	F value	P value	Freq.	Mean	SD	DoF	F value	P value
They are trying hard	36	4.5	0.845	1	0.396	0.532	69	4.35	0.968	1	0.315	0.576
	29	4.34	1.143	63			47	4.45	0.88	114		
I miss them	34	4.62	0.697	1	0.329	0.568	66	4.47	0.845	1	1.143	0.287
	29	4.52	0.688	61			48	4.63	0.64	112		
I feel sorry for them	34	3.97	1.141	1	0.124	0.726	61	3.89	1.142	1	0.951	0.332
	29	3.86	1.302	61			46	4.09	0.939	105		
I feel bad for leaving	32	2.81	1.447	1	2.13	0.15	60	3.05	1.383	1	5.025	0.027
	29	3.34	1.396	59			46	3.63	1.236	104		
I understand	32	4	0.88	1	0.148	0.701	62	4	0.905	1	0	1
	29	3.9	1.205	59			47	4	0.885	107		
They should evacuate	32	3.56	1.014	1	0.564	0.456	64	3.42	1.081	1	4.54	0.035
	29	3.76	1.023	59			47	3.83	0.868	109		
It's uncomfortable	29	2.38	1.347	1	0.513	0.477	60	2.38	1.209	1	10.523	0.002
	29	2.14	1.217	56			47	3.17	1.291	105		
I want to help	33	3.52	1.121	1	8.556	0.005	62	4	1.04	1	1.964	0.164
	29	4.31	1.004	60			47	4.26	0.793	107		

Note: Top values correspond to those not living with children aged 12 and under, bottom values correspond to those who are.

III. Examination

1. Severity of the situation

The lives of a great many people were drastically transformed by the 2011 off the Pacific coast of Tohoku earthquake, subsequent tsunami, and the nuclear power plant accident that followed. Particularly in regard to the nuclear power plant accident, the disaster has gone beyond the level of temporary disaster to become a major problem that will continue to threaten the health and even the very lives of people for decades. This survey has provided us with a look at the severity of the situation the families of Tohoku, and particularly those forced to flee from Fukushima, have found themselves in. Families have been broken apart, have moved repeatedly and frequently, and even a year after the disaster, the foundation on which theirs lives are built remains unstable, and their prospects for the future remain unclear. It is as if they have been deprived of the right to life guaranteed by the Japanese constitution.

The separation of spouses and fathers from their children was deemed particularly serious. A comprehensive look at the results suggests that these families may have been broken up when mothers fled with their children in order to protect them from the harm caused by the radiation released during the nuclear power plant accident and left their husbands behind. It is reasonable to assume that these separations occurred as a result of fathers remaining behind in the affected regions in order to keep working. Continuing to live in this sort of situation lacks stability, but there is little prospect of these families returning to Tohoku in the near future, leaving them at a loss.

In this way, evacuee families have been forced to suffer much, separated from direct family members and other relatives, separated from and deprived of the communities and lands they come from, and required to enter new communities and lands and adapt to the customs and people. Negayama, et al. (2012) considered the lives of evacuee families to be in a state of transition, with the process moving from ① securing survival, to ② maintaining the foundations of livelihood, and ③ finding life perspective for the future. This study was conducted less than one year after the earthquake. By that time, the evacuees had transitioned from the "escape with the clothes on their backs, just find shelter" stage of the evacuation, and moved into the stage during which they were seeking out a more stable living environment, and to a certain extent, their lives had begun to calm down at last. In that sense, they were in the transition between stages ① and ②.

At the time, Negayama, et al. (2012) posited that there were signs of people reorganizing their lives and transitioning from stage ② to stage ③, and that new issues were beginning to arise, including stress due to isolation from the community networks and normalized separation from others, fixed estrangement, etc. Although two years have passed since then, currently (in 2014), it is difficult to say that there have been any major improvements in conditions. While some families have managed to fit in with their new communities and almost rebuild their lives, other families have found the extent of their difficulties deepen. In fact, there are also concerns such difficulties will continue to increase as the disparities between families become greater. The poverty of national policies today seems to be reflected here. At the same time, it is also sad that the disaster is now being gradually forgotten by the forgetful society as a past event in spite of, at the time of the disaster, support from around the country to deal with that unprecedented tragedy.

As will be explained in the next section, mothers are prone to long-term negative effects caused by the nuclear power plant accident. This study also found that mothers who evacuated with small children without their spouses had significantly strongly negative psychological issues. In a later questionnaire study (as yet unpublished), we again confirmed that there was a significant correlation between stress in children from evacuee families and maternal stress. It goes without saying that careful attention must be paid to this issue in the future, particularly regarding relationships between mothers and small children.

However, at the same time, as parents have a strong sense of responsibility regarding their children, it cannot be ruled out that they saw the nuclear power plant accident as severe and stressful and fled to Kanto with their children. Unless we also consider alternatives to such causality of "the nuclear power plant accident → radiation injury → evacuation → stress," we may come to an incorrect conclusion.

2. Other research

There have been three major nuclear catastrophes in the last thirty years or so – a meltdown at Three Mile Island in the USA in 1979, an uncontrolled explosive reaction at Chernobyl in the USSR in 1986, and the disaster at Fukushima in 2011. In terms of human history, it would be appropriate to state that they are frequent. Once nuclear power gets uncontrolled, according to current knowledge, it is extremely difficult to restore the control of it. Moreover, the severity of a nuclear disaster is unparalleled, in pathological and geographical terms, and in terms of the time required to clean it up.

Bromet and others have conducted valuable research and provided valuable suggestions regarding the physical and mental impact of nuclear accidents with follow-up studies on the accidents at Three Mile Island (Bromet, et al., 1982; Dew and Bromet, 1993), Chernobyl (Bromet, et al., 2002; Bromet and Havenaar, 2007), and even Fukushima (Bromet, 2014). They reported that their research found a profound effect on workers engaged in post-accident cleanup on site and on mothers with children living nearby, but that children themselves were resilient.

As mentioned above, we continue to conduct support-based research through the *Kasasagi* Project for two purposes. First, since the unprecedented disaster resulted in an infringement of the fundamental human rights of victims guaranteed by the Japanese constitution, we as fellows will use our know-how to help improve that situation. Also, more specifically, it allows us, who have considered how to separate children from parents healthily under the keyword "*Kowakare* (mother-child separation)," to look at how children in Japanese families and communities develop after living through the separations and difficulties faced by their families. For that reason, we are not only engaged in this research, but also in observation and interviews of evacuee families, and more recently, in other activities that include helping hold gatherings for evacuee families, helping evacuee children create puppet plays, and more.

3. Future issues

Evacuee families were separated from their hometowns and interpersonal networks and forced to move to new areas and join new interpersonal networks. They have to look towards their futures and rebuild their lives. The future of the nuclear power plant is unclear and society's interest has waned, so it will be difficult to settle on an outlook for life. We must continue to reach out and provide support when needed to people working on these issues. When we do so, we need a correct understanding of the complex situations and diverse needs of people involved, and need to make the effort to empower such individuals to make the choices they need to make on their own.

In addition, we believe that, as developmental scientists, we must monitor the developmental effects of such severe conditions on children who experience them in infancy and early childhood. However, we must not simply look at how they are negatively influenced or whether or not they are able to bear the burden. We must take the multifaceted view and consider what sort of "benefits" such an experience has and what sort of "positive" influences can occur. We must consider the issue over the long-term.

Three years after the earthquake, we should now turn our gaze to society, which is forgetting the disaster. When our fellows are facing the difficulties being forced to live deprived of fundamental human rights, in order to encourage people to accept the issue as shared problem that requires support, we must continue raising these questions and raising their awareness within society.

Acknowledgements

This research was first made possible through the cooperation of the evacuee families, but also through the cooperation of the Shinsai Shien Network Saitama (represented by Tadashi Inomata), everyone working on the Waseda University's Disaster and Human Science Project (represented by Takuya Tsujiuchi and Kazutaka Masuda), and all of the people in the related departments of the municipalities of Saitama Prefecture. Moreover, we received funding from the Japan Psychological Association Tohoku Earthquake Reconstruction Fund for Practical and Research Activities (Support for network formation and related activities among evacuee children); a Meiji Yasuda Mental Health Foundation Grant (Examining desirable methods of empowering evacuee families); the Waseda University Tohoku Earthquake Reconstruction Research Hub Short-term Research Project (Supporting parents and children separated by the disaster) (all represented by Koichi Negayama). We would like to express our appreciation to all these financial supports here.

References

Bromet, E. J., 2014. Emotional consequences of nuclear power plant disasters. *Health Physics*, 106, 206-210.

Bromet, E.J., Gluzman, S., Schwartz, J.E., Goldgaber, D., 2002. Somatic symptoms in women 11 years after the Chernobyl accident. *Environmental Health Perspectives*, 110 (Supplement 4), 625-629.

Bromet, E. J., Havenaar, J.M., 2007. Psychological and perceived health effects of the Chernobyl disaster: a 20-year review. *Health Physics*, 93, 516-521.

Bromet, E.J., Havenaar, J.M., Guey, L.T., 2011. A 25 year retrospective review of the psychological consequences of the Chernobyl accident. *Clinical Oncology*, 23, 297-305.

Bromet, E. J., Parkinson, D. K., Schulberg, H. C., Dunn, L. O., Gondek, P. C., 1982. Mental health of residents near the Three Mile Island reactor: a comparative study of selected groups. *Journal of Preventive Psychiatry*, 1, 225-275.

Cherry, K. E., 2009. Life-span Perspectives on Natural Disasters: Coping with Katrina, Rita, and Other Storms, Springer.

Dew, M. A., Bromet, E.J., 1998. Predictors of temporal patterns of psychiatric distress during 10 years following the nuclear accident at Three Mile Island. *Social Psychiatry and Psychiatric Epidemiology*, 28, 49-55.

Hirata, S., Ishijima, K., Mochida, R., Negayama, K., 2013. *Shinsai hinan kazoku no shien – kasasagi purojekuto no katsudō*. [Supporting families evacuating earthquakes: activities of the *Kasasagi* Project.], In: Tsujiuchi, T. (Ed.), *Gajyumaru teki shien no susume – hitori hitori no kokoro ni yorisou: Higashi nihon daishinsai to ningen kagaku 1.* [The Great East Japan Earthquake and Human Science 1: Recommendations of Banyan-like Support – Getting closer to each individual.], Waseda University Booklet, After the Disaster 31, Waseda University Press, pp. 17-39.

Hirata, S., Negayama, K., Ishijima, K., Mochida, R., Shiraga, A., 2012. *Kasasagi purojekuto ni yoru shinsai hinan kazoku no shien.* [Support for families forced to live separately due to the Fukushima nuclear disaster: an interim report of the *Kasasagi* Project.], *Human Science Research*, 25 (2), 265-272.

Masten, A. S., Narayan, A.J., 2011. Child development in the context of disaster, war, and terrorism: pathways of risk and resilience, *Annual Review of Psychology*, 63, 227-257.

Masten, A. S., Osofsky J. D., 2010. Disasters and their impact on child development: introduction to the special section. *Child Development*, 81, 1029-1039.

Negayama, K., 2010. *Kyōdai jishin eno taiō ni mirareru oyako kankei – kowakare no kanten kara no kentō.* [Reactions of children and parents to an earthquake, from the viewpoint of 'Kowakare' (Mutual autonomy).], *The Japanese Journal of Developmental Psychology*, 21, 386-395.

Negayama, K., Hirata, S., Ishijima, K., 2012. *Genpatsu jiko ni yoru hinan kazoku eno shien.* [Support for families forced to live separately due to the Fukushima nuclear disaster.], *Japanese Journal of Clinical Developmental Psychology*, 7, 42-46.

7 Mental Health / Family Health / Community Health

How Evacuee Families with Children Adapt

Considering relationships with their communities

Shuzo Hirata MA [1] *(Developmental Psychology, Child Welfare),*
Konomi Ishijima MA [2][6] *(Developmental psychology),*
Ryuhei Mochida MA [3] *(Developmental psychology),*
Yuko Shiraishi MA [4] *(Developmental psychology),*
Koichi Negayama PhD [5][6] *(Developmental Human Ethology)*

Key words: nuclear power plant accident, voluntary evacuation, community network, case study, Kasasagi Project

I. Introduction

On the 11th of March 2011, a massive, magnitude-9 earthquake, the Tohoku Earthquake, struck the Tohoku area, setting off a complex series of disasters that included a tsunami and nuclear power plant accident that all combine to force many to evacuate their homes. According to a 2014 report by the Reconstruction Agency, there were 243,040 evacuees by September 2014, three and a half years after the disaster, 30,405 of whom had evacuated to the Kanto area.

The authors of this paper belong to the Developmental Ethology Laboratory at Waseda University's Faculty of Human Sciences, where since June 2011, we have been working on the *Kasasagi* Project to survey and support families that evacuated to Kanto after the disaster. The project is involved in a diverse range of activities, but from the very beginning, it has been particularly focused on families that were split

---

[1] Lecturer, Department of Child Studies, Sendai Seiyo Gakuin College
[2] Research Associate, Department of Education for Childcare, Tokyo Kasei University
[3] Visiting Researcher, Advanced Research Center for Human Sciences, Waseda University
[4] Research Fellow, Center for Brain Science, Institute of Physical and Chemical Research (RIKEN)
[5] Professor, Faculty of Human Sciences, Waseda University
[6] Waseda Institute of Medical Anthropology on Disaster Reconstruction (WIMA)

apart when mothers and children evacuated to Kanto, leaving fathers behind at home. This sort of case is thought to be a common one among the families that evacuated. From November 2011 to January 2012, a questionnaire survey targeting evacuees in Saitama Prefecture was conducted (See Negayama, et al., Paper #30 in this publication). That survey uncovered that large numbers of mothers evacuated with their children from areas outside of the designated evacuation zones, and the results showed a clear trend of families among which the fathers remained behind while the children evacuated with their mothers to avoid radiation injury.

In addition, because the mothers had evacuated voluntarily with their children, there was a delay in understanding the makeup of the evacuees as a group, and government response and support often did not reach the evacuees, especially during the period shortly after the disaster. Many families experienced difficulties, with children deprived of their fathers, fathers deprived of their children, and spouses deprived of each other's company. Moreover, mothers and children had to face changes in their living environment, as they were separated from their old community networks and forced to migrate to new communities. Families were forced to respond to these issues in various ways that were difficult to bear, and also had to deal with them for a long period of time (Hirata, et al., 2012).

The following presents the objective and significance of this paper which takes the above facts into consideration. First, this paper provides case studies of two families of mothers who evacuated with their children who were studied and supported by the authors. Particular attention was paid to the sense of crisis and friction family members felt regarding relationships inside and outside of the family both during and after the evacuation, and how they adapted to their new environments. The paper also examines how that changed moment to moment over time in connection with the conditions faced. Through that, the paper aims to provide a detailed view of one side of the process through which mothers and children who evacuated adapted to their post-earthquake lives while facing various situations, and at the same time, aims to gain a perspective regarding the form support should take. Other researchers who have qualitatively studied the living conditions of mothers who evacuated with their children include Konno & Sato (2014) and Yamane (2013). What sets this study apart from those is that it continued from June 2011 until now in 2014, and aimed to gain an understanding of the overall process from immediately after the evacuation to the current day.

Portions of the information in this paper have appeared in other papers by the authors (Hirata, et al., 2012, Hirata, et al., 2013, Negayama, et al., 2012), and while some information overlaps, it has been rewritten for this paper in relation to the progress thereafter.

II. Method: Surveying and supporting evacuee mothers and children through the *Kasasagi* Project

1. Meeting up with evacuee mothers and children

In June 2011, the authors were put in touch with five families of evacuee mothers and children (evacuee families below) by a former graduate student who was living in Fukushima Prefecture, and we interviewed them regarding their experiences with the earthquake. Then proposals were made regarding potential support of the authors, and the continuous survey thereafter was asked for.

The following support was proposed/implemented for the evacuee families, and includes activities only conducted immediately after evacuating when conditions were in a constant state of flux. However, of course these forms of support did not necessarily fulfill all of the needs of the evacuees, and not all evacuee families even wanted the support the authors could provide. As a result, the authors are currently in regular contact with two families as of October 2014. The families who didn't wish to take part in the survey or receive support were informed that if they experienced any difficulties the authors were available for consultation at any time.

2. Support details

-Played outside with the children, who had had few chances to play with their friends immediately after evacuating, and let the mothers have a break in the meantime.
-Provided computers and other devices installed with Skype to allow the evacuee families to have face-to-face contact their husbands/fathers.
-Provided support to the Evacuee Families Group (described below) launched by the evacuee families themselves.
-Gave feedback on the survey and provided counselling on child care and other topics. (Also informed the families that clinical psychologists were available for consultation.)

3. Survey method/ethical considerations

The following were also implemented in order to gain a comprehensive understanding as much as possible of the constantly changing conditions the evacuee families found themselves in, and to be able to respond flexibly through support and other means. The survey/support process can be described as a form of "action research" (Hosaka, 2003), which is based on the process through which researchers and practitioners mutually influence each other. This survey was conducted after reporting to the Waseda University Ethics Committee.
-Interviews conducted during multiple visits to where the evacuee families were living (from June 2011)
-Interviews with fathers in Fukushima (November 2011, February 2013)

-Monitoring and recording of child activity levels in their new environments through video camera/GPS/Actigraph(an activity monitoring device)

III. Results and Examination: Through the cases of two evacuee families

Two families (Family A and Family B) which have been surveyed and provided with support from June 2011 up to the current time in 2014. Among their narratives, observations of them and other episodes, we discussed the sense of crisis and friction family members felt regarding relationships within the family and with people outside of each family both during and after the evacuation, and how they adapted to their new environments. This information was collated in chronological order and displayed as a function of time. Table 1 shows the overall findings.

Narrative boxes containing excerpts of conversations with the families are found throughout this paper. Text in (round brackets) signifies a question from the researchers, the term "omitted" signifies that a part of the person's statement has been removed, and text in [square brackets] indicates information that has been added by the authors. Underlined text is used to provide the appropriate explanations.

1. Immediately after evacuation until March 2012

(1) Differences in opinion between spouses, parents and children, and other relatives when forced to choose

Rumors flew rampant after the March 11 earthquake and subsequent nuclear accident, and as the situation continued to change constantly, families were continually forced to make new decisions in response. This led to cases of differing judgement and even conflict between spouses, between parents and children, and with other relatives.

Mother A: My husband kept saying he was going to work anyway even after the hydrogen explosion, and I guess I kind of felt, 'should I really be married to this guy?' (Mother A laughs.) I thought that we should first be evacuating as a family. For a time I was angry at him because I didn't know what to do. (June 2011)

Mother B: We didn't tell my husband parents [that we were voluntarily evacuating]. (Omitted) We didn't live very far away from each other, but we didn't talk often. (Omitted) It was tough. It was a generational difference. Lots of people just don't understand why someone would evacuate. They understand if it's the national government or the prefectural government telling someone to do it though. There's lots of people like that. For example, since someone's mother-in-law doesn't understand, she cannot leave. (July 2011)

How Evacuee Families with Children Adapt 203

Mother A explained how directly after the nuclear power plant accident she and her husband had different opinions about what to do; she felt the family should evacuate together, while her husband felt that he should prioritize work. The couple later discussed the situation and decided that the husband would evacuate his wife and children to Kanto and he would return alone to Fukushima. Mother A knew that other families were unable to evacuate due to the husband's opposition, which made her appreciate her husband even more, and their bond as a couple actually grew stronger.

Mother B said that she was concerned that her relatives wouldn't understand why she wanted to voluntarily evacuate to Kanto, and she said initially hesitated to tell them. There were apparently no large issues when her relatives learned that Family B had voluntarily evacuated. However, after initially evacuating, she was concerned that her relatives would disagree with her decision. We should consider this carefully, because such concern could lead the evacuees to feel guilty about evacuating, or feel that they had made it more difficult for the relatives to help each other out.

Fortunately, neither Family A nor Family B experienced any major issues within their families or with other relatives, and there were even cases in which relationships grew stronger. However, depending on the family, in some cases in which such difference of opinion arises, they may not be able to close the gap between them.

Table 1. Experience of evacuee families (Family A and Family B)

	Evacuee Families (Family A & Family B)	
1 Earthquake until end of March 2012	(1) Differences in opinion between spouses, parents and children, and other relatives when forced to choose (2) Loneliness due to separation (3) Complicated mentality regarding old and new relationships (4) Establishment of Evacuee Families Group (5) Future unclear - "Up in the air" (6) Children expressing their stress (7) Child resilience and passivity in adapting to new communities after evacuating	
2 From April 2012	Family reunited in Kanto (Family A)	Mother and children remain evacuated (Family B)
	(1) Relief and confusion after reunited (2) Fluctuating self-recognition: "We are evacuees." "We are not evacuees." (3) Reorganizing relationships (4) Child's best friend is a friend from Fukushima	(5) Difficulty for family to find time to relax and talk together (6) Continued uncertainty regarding future, and difficulties dealing with that (7) Friction between families that did evacuate from non-designated evacuations areas and those that didn't

(2) Loneliness due to separation
In both Family A and Family B, fathers in Fukushima remained in frequent phone contact with their wives and children in Kanto and visited their families once or twice

a month, but every member of each family was made to feel a sense of loneliness due to the separation.

> Mother A: My son often looks like he's trying not to cry. Even when we say goodbye (when his father is about to return to Fukushima after a visit with the family)…at first he cried all the time. (June 2011)

In addition to the separation from the father, this loneliness seems to have been spurred on by having been pulled away from the community and people they were used to, and the lack of clarity regarding the future. Father A also complained about the loneliness he felt living alone long-term away from his family.

(3) Complicated mentality regarding old and new relationships

> Mother A: I feel sorry about the friends back there…it's hard to stay in touch. I can only really talk with other friends who ran away here. Having said that, I have friends in my hometown [Tokyo], but no matter who I meet, I can't just spend all my time talking about the thing I'm most worried about, the radiation, and other things about me. (Omitted) It's like, I think something about me has changed… it kind of hurts. (Omitted) Everyone around here is really open and friendly. And I'm really thankful for that… (Omitted) But when things start to calm down, we have fewer and fewer chances to meet. (Omitted) I might only be here for six months…there's that too. (Omitted) I think they are trying to be friendly, but I think maybe the only people I can talk about my real feelings with are other friends who went through the same experience as me. (June 2011)
>
> Mother B: I'm not really comfortable with other mothers yet. (She laughs.) Can I call them friends? It's always in the morning, the kids gather to go to school together, and everyone has to go downstairs. The mothers all have to come out too [gather in the plaza in front of the condominium to send the children off to school]. It's like, they all do their makeup before they come down in the morning …I just can't do that. (She laughs.) (July 2011)

In Mother A's narrative, she describes her feelings in regard to four different types of relationships (as underlined above): friends back there (i.e. friends left behind in Fukushima); friends who ran away here (i.e. friends who evacuated from Fukushima to Kanto); friends in her hometown (i.e. friends already in Kanto); and everyone around here (i.e. the people who live in the community to which she and her family evacuated). Her narrative shows that she seems to have created deeper bonds with the friends who also evacuated from Fukushima to Kanto, although she feels guilty about leaving other friends behind in Fukushima. Moreover, she also seems to be hesitating when it comes to forging new relationships with those in the community she lives in now. Looking at it from a more serious perspective, it is possible that Mother A felt that she emotionally isolated in the community to which she evacuated, but we also see that she may have felt mutually anchored by the friendships she had with other people who also evacuated from Fukushima.

In Mother B's narrative, she describes the initial embarrassment she felt at the customs in her new community. She laughs as she describes her issue, suggesting that she isn't taking the problem as a serious one, but more attention is paid to evacuees in new communities than would be paid were they simply new to the neighborhood, and as support is provided by those around the evacuees, this difference in customs could potentially cause a significant amount of stress in an individual.

(4) Establishment of Evacuee Families Group

Mother A and Mother B were behind the launch of the Evacuee Families Group in July 2011. Members were primarily evacuee mothers and children in the Kanto area, and around 15 people initially participated. We spoke to the mothers about the establishment of the group and their motivation for activities to get a more detailed understanding of the circumstances behind its launch.

(Do you ever wish there was other forms of help available to you?)

Mother A: Right now, it's actually less that I want help... I also lived in Fukushima for five years, and I'm starting to see something...I feel somewhat ashamed. I want to help reclaim the soil in Fukushima. And help build a network that makes Fukushima people safer. (Omitted) I want to do that. I know there's nothing really that I can do, but that's the sort of thing I want to do. (Omitted) I want to get into the position where I can support others as quickly as I can. (June 2011)

This conversation took place immediately after things began to calm down for Family A's evacuation. Here, we see a voluntary evacuee hesitant to describe herself as "someone needing support." She also talks about a feeling of shame in regard to her old community, and an earnest desire to take it upon herself to help start the reconstruction in Fukushima. It is thought that the feelings she describes above, along with the complicated mentality regarding old and new relationships as previously discussed, had a large influence on the launch of the Evacuee Families Group. Moreover, the members of the mother's group frequently participated in meetings regarding the nuclear plant and compensation. This suggests they have a strong motivation to communicate to the rest of society the conditions in which they as voluntary evacuees were living.

The authors initially arranged the venue for the inaugural meeting and helped the mothers create a venue that was easy for them to gather in. However, after seeing and hearing about the development of the Evacuee Families Group which was launched in such a way, the authors were given a new look at the minds and strength of the evacuee mothers, and afterwards, the entire stance of the project was adjusted. In specific terms, rather than define it in terms of "supporter and supported" it was decided that the project would study the voluntary evacuees as proactive communicators and as people living proactive lives, all the while remaining available to provide quick help should a problem arise.

(5) Future unclear – "Up in the air"
During visits with the mothers and children, the authors were given a glimpse into how they felt at different moments, but after passing the three-month mark since their evacuation, the mothers began to speak particularly often about a feeling of being left unsettled, through comments such as "We're just up in the air…everything is vague" or "We can't move on" and "If I can't find a job, we'll have no future." The families had managed to surmount the imminent danger through evacuation, and secured an autonomous environment in which to live, but they had also begun looking towards the future, to finding work and their overall long-term lives and lifestyle prospects.

(6) Children expressing their stress
Post-evacuation life for Family A began to settle down in around May or June 2011, and Mother A became aware of some behavioral issues with her children.

> Mother A: About a month ago [around May], physically <u>my son</u> started to…I don't know how to explain it…he started doing this (she makes a chewing motion with her mouth). (Omitted) I started thinking that must be psychological…like a type of tic or something. (Omitted) With elevators too, he absolutely refused to ride them alone because if there was an earthquake it would stop. (Omitted) Recently, <u>my daughter</u> started saying…about a week ago…that her throat hurts. (Omitted) We went to the pediatrician, who just said, "There's absolutely nothing wrong."
>
> That symptom seems to be gone, but now she complains every day, "My stomach hurts. MY stomach hurts." (June 2011)

Family A have two children, a boy of seven and a girl of three (at the time of the disaster). The description above suggests that, after life began to settle down after evacuation, the following things may have occurred with the children.

First, there were tic-like symptoms, which are considered to be a physical indicator of stress and tension, and a continued fear of earthquake even after they had evacuated. In addition, the three-year-old daughter's behavior of frequent complaints to her mother, particularly from the point of view of a young child, could have arisen from the fact that her parents' decisions had constantly changed situations, from the earthquake to the evacuation, and they hadn't had enough time to spend with their children. Thus, the child may have been attempting to get her mother's attention once things began to settle down, or to a certain extent, may have been expressing a form of dissatisfaction.

(7) Child resilience and passivity in adapting to new communities after evacuating
To understand how the children of Family A and Family B were adapting to live in their new communities post-evacuation, the authors conducted a comprehensive study based on the narratives of the mothers and fathers, and on the results of our observations conducted on the children. Initially, the children were forced to go to schools in their new communities and build new relationships without sufficient preparation, but it was concluded that two behavioral aspects could be observed: both a strong effort to blend in, and lack of motivation to blend in (June to November 2011).

Examples of the former were observed when neighborhood children were playing with water outside. One of the children saw one of the members of this project standing apart from everyone else and got suspicious. Then the child shared the suspicion with the evacuee child, who then splashed the project member with water. Later, when the children said goodbye to each other, the evacuee child had a very guilty look. (⇒It is thought that the child was still uncertain about their acceptance into the neighborhood group of children, and took the chance to participate in the group by joining in with treating the project member as an enemy.) Another example had one child attempting to contact friends in the disaster area over the internet. Examples of the latter could be observed when one of the project members was playing outside with an evacuee child, and another child of about the same age passed by. The evacuee child looked at the other child, seemed to want to approach, but didn't take the first step. Other information was gathered by GPS and Actigraph, the data from which showed a tendency towards little activity and movement.

Regarding the passiveness about being accepted, the mother described that the child seemed to be overwhelmed about something during the first semester of school. Also, [at first] she'd talked about returning to Fukushima in six months, and felt that she shouldn't try and get close to the other mothers in the neighborhood. The mother guessed that her son may have taken on some of those same feelings from her. It is possible that the child had little emotional energy to spare, or perhaps indirectly reflected the complex mental state of the parents.

As described above, in the examples of the children of Family A and Family B in adapting to their new communities, apparently they either attempted to do so with an understanding of their own position and while monitoring the people and situation around them, or hesitated to blend in entirely. This seems to have been closely related to the overall uncertainty regarding the future for the families.

2. From April 2012

Here we discuss the example of the family that reunited in Kanto and the family for which the mother and children remained evacuated.

Case: Family A reunites in Kanto

(1) Relief and confusion after reunited

Family A was reunited in 2012 when Father A relocated to Kanto. The following narrative was provided during a visit after things had settled down after the move following the relocation.

> Mother A: At first I tried to be careful and align myself with how my husband was living, (Omitted) and I had wanted us to get back together as quickly as we could while we were evacuated, but I just felt like he was in the way [once they started living together again]. (Omitted) But I think he had a lot of stress. I think he might have been stressed out about me as well. (Omitted)
> •
> Did anything change for your children after their father arrived? They must have been happy.)
>
> Mother A: Sure, they were happy. Basically. But…(Omitted) Once or twice my son told me that he thought it had been better when it was just the three of us, and I'd said something like that as well just before that, so even though it felt that he was just copying what I said, I was rather shocked to hear it come from his mouth. But I realized it was something I'd said, and I felt a bit sorry about it. (August 2012)

This narrative does not include detailed descriptions of the feelings of all family members, but although they had been waiting for the time when they could live together as a family again, but once they were reunited, the members of the family seem to have been subject to some stress. When the family was living separately, with father on one side and mother and children on the other, they would have created a new system to adapt to the situation. It is possible that once the family was reunited, that system had to be reorganized again, and this caused a temporary period of instability. Psychologically speaking, it creates an almost contradictory emotional environment that lies somewhere between relief and confusion.

In the case of Family A, the authors visited again in September 2014 to inquire about conditions then, and the family answered that "it's no different than before the earthquake," so it seems that they fortunately were able to return to a more stable state. That being said, changes in the family system can result in a form of crisis. Had a large conflict emerged while the father was living apart from the mother and children, the period of instability after they were reunited may have continued long term, and potentially could have resulted in an emotional backlash.

(2) Fluctuating self-recognition: "We are evacuees." "We are not evacuees."

(How did you feel when you decided to build a future in Kanto?)

Mother A: I am so indebted to the people around here... it almost hurts. (Omitted) I wanted us to be independent, so I felt a bit relieved as well. Yes. (Omitted) But I helped launch the Evacuee Families Group, and I participated in it with my friends. And now it feels like I'm the only one who isn't an evacuee anymore. (Omitted) I think I might have a bit depressed about it for the first month or so... (August 2012)

For Mother A, defining herself as an "evacuee" meant that she recognized that she was someone who needed the help and support of others. Regarding that indebtedness she described it as if "it almost hurts," so once her family was reunited and they began to live independently again, she felt "relieved." On the other hand, while she was still recognized as "one of them" by the friends she had made among the other evacuees during her evacuation life, she remained conscious of that relationship, and her own self-recognition had begun to waver. That fluctuation in self-recognition is thought to be closely connected to the content in the next section: Reorganizing relationships.

(3) Reorganizing relationships
This section is not compiled from interviews recorded with the members of Families A and B, but rather from the record of conversation between the authors and the evacuees including the members of Families A and B (the field notes). The lifestyles of evacuees continue to diverge and diversify, and at this point in 2014, this is considered to be an important thing faced by the evacuees, so it was thought appropriate to include this section here.

As discussed in the sections, "Complicated mentality regarding old and new relationships" and "Establishment of Evacuee Families Group," evacuees from outside the designated evacuation zones had to adapt while they experienced some complicated feelings regarding the friends and relatives who decided to remain in Fukushima and regarding their neighbors in the communities to which they had evacuated. There also was observed a movement towards solidarity among the evacuees with shared experiences. However, as time passed, the lives the evacuees chose to take diversified, with some deciding to reunite in Kanto, some leaving the father in Fukushima while they continued to live in Kanto, some returning to Fukushima, and more. This diversification can have an effect on the relationships the evacuees have built with each other since the evacuation.

In Mother A's case, she spoke about a period during which she started thinking about whether or not it was appropriate for her to continue to participate in the Evacuee Families Group when she began to wonder whether she saw herself as an evacuee or not (March 2013). However, at the time of the interview in September 2014, her relationships with her "friends from the Evacuee Families Group" had continued, and she rather considered them to be friends who had shared the experience of the earthquake and the evacuation. She described it, saying "I feel most at ease when I'm with them, I don't have to pretend to be someone I'm not, and we always have fun together." She described that those feelings have grown stronger, and that she now feels she is where she belongs. In addition, her previous worries regarding whether or not she belonged in the group were eased completely when one of her friends in the Evacuee Families Group told her that she was "not an evacuee, but someone who experienced the evacuation."

In other words, we can see how the evacuees connected to Mother A are now beginning to build relationships without being concerned about the different positions people occupy. The rebuilding and maintenance of these relationships suggests that the women see their having evacuated as an important shared experience. However, this may not always be the case when we consider this from the perspective of evacuees as a whole. Therefore, future research must look in greater detail into the specific aspects of these reconstructed relationships, including the relationships built in the communities to which these individuals evacuated.

(4) Child's best friend is a friend from Fukushima
The authors conducted interviews with the mothers in August 2013 and September 2014 to inquire about the relationships the children had built. Family A's son (who was seven at the time of the disaster) made new friends in Kanto, but had no one he could call a best friend, telling his mother that, "My best friend is still XX in Fukushima." The two children apparently still meet once or twice a year. Childhood is the period during which relationships develop, so perhaps the son still sees the relation-

ship with his best friend in Fukushima as very important, but the truth behind what this narrative means remains unclear and should be the subject of future detailed study.

Family B Mother and child remain evacuated
(5) Difficulty for family to find time to relax and talk together
As of November 2014, Father B remains alone in Fukushima while his wife and child live as evacuees. His son (nine at the time of the disaster) currently attends a junior high school in Kanto, and the current living conditions are expected to continue for the time being.

> Father B: Whenever we (as spouses) talk about [living conditions in the future], [son] listens really carefully, ears perked, behind us somewhere as mom and dad talk. And yeah, he is really worried about that, and it's naturally something he cares about. That's who he is. That's why I don't know if we should try to talk about it as little as possible, or if we should be completely open about it and talk about it as a family. There is such a sort of thing. Right now I'm trying to be a bit more careful, and not really talk about specifics.
> ●
> I don't ever have time to just sit down and relax and talk with him [his son]. When I go there [where his wife and son live] I try as often as possible to take him to a public bath or that sort of thing, maybe to a foot bath. Somewhere we can have a chance to talk. (February 2013)

In Family B, the father usually visits his wife and son in Kanto about once a month, and the mother and son return to the home in Fukushima during longer vacations and other chances. In addition, Father B calls his wife and son every morning, so they all wake up together, and he calls again at night when his son returns from cram schools. What this narrative first shows us is that when the mother and father discuss the future and the like at such times, their son listens carefully nearby out of worry. We also learn that Father B is conscious of this, and attempts to avoid the conversation with his wife, while at the same time, proactively creating opportunities to speak with his son.

The evacuation of the mother and son meant that the family's time together is limited, but because of that, they should try to make the most of the time they do spend together. That makes it easier to understand why the family seems to have fostered an atmosphere in which they try to avoid more serious topics, such as the subject of their future living situation. In addition, a situation in which it is more difficult to picture what the future should be seems to further promote such an atmosphere.

(6) Continued uncertainty regarding future, and difficulties dealing with that

> Father B: The situation now makes me worry about what we'll do in the future. It's like nothing is clear. (Omitted) Maybe they'll come home next year...no... [son] has started junior high school there [in the community to which they evacuated] so he'd have to graduate first before coming home...or maybe not. That's the thing. That's the thing I just really don't know what to do about. (Omitted) Because it's not like [the deemed temporary housing system] will last forever. And obviously we can't have the house here and rent an apartment down there. We'll be at the point where we really have to make a decision about it. (February 2013)
>
> Mother B: I still don't know what's going to happen next. Everything's up in the air. We get more exhausted the longer it lasts too. We can't stay evacuated forever. Recently I've started thinking about how long we're going to end up being evacuees for. (February 2013)

Father B and Mother B were interviewed at around the same time in different locations, and both expressed a shared feeling of concern about their unclear future, and it seemed that their son's academic progress and the deemed temporary housing system were issues deeply related to that worry. This situation is thought to be applicable to many evacuees. The feeling of being "up in the air" have still continued since the interview conducted three months after the evacuation. That had caused the family to become fatigued, and the family were all aware of it.

(7) Friction between families that did evacuate from non-designated evacuations areas and those that didn't

> Father B: I'll go to the local commerce and industry gatherings and people will say, "Hey, your family's still running away?" When people start drinking, that's all they talk about. (Omitted) I mean, I understand where they're coming from. (Omitted) They have employees, and if they had their children and wives living somewhere else, I don't know if that would work. (Omitted) I think a part of it is having made that really difficult choice. (Omitted) That kind of thing will come up. Naturally. Everything's complicated. (February 2013)

Father B remains in Fukushima and his narrative shows that there were various factors at play behind a decision about whether or not to evacuate in areas not designated as evacuation zones, and that there are cases where this has become a source of some discord between those whose families evacuated and those whose families remained. It is thought that this will also have a large effect on the evacuees' decisions about whether or not to return to Fukushima in the future.

IV. Summary

This research has shown that evacuee mothers with children who independently made the decision to voluntarily evacuate immediately after the earthquake to Kanto have experienced various crisis and friction in their relationships with others both inside and outside of the families. Overall, it also illustrates the process through which people powerfully adapt. Simultaneously, this research clarified that families in which the mothers and children are still evacuated get more fatigued with little clarity about the future, while families that have reunited experience a period of instability immediately after reintegrating, and interpersonal relationships with those inside and outside of the family can be reorganized.

It is thought that few reunited families are viewed as "evacuees" by others. However, families that experienced differences in opinion between spouses, parents and children, and other relatives when forced to choose during evacuation or while evacuated may unexpectedly see a major crisis unfold. Naturally, most families will likely not experience that, but considering the appearance of the term "genpatsu rikon" (or nuclear plant divorce), even once families are no longer evacuees, it would seem necessary to take great care.

For families still living life as evacuee mothers and children, there is some concern about the various problems they face and the fatigue that has accumulated while facing those problems. As described here, it is thought that the lack of clear prospects for the future may have a large influence on this, but as the housing provision system for evacuees and the free highway travel system for evacuee families are subject to annual renewal, it is difficult to visualize any long-term prospects there. National policy itself has a direct influence on the conditions in which evacuee families live. This should also be heavily related to the financial background of evacuee families. As Conger and Donnellan(2007) insisted that economic distress can trigger emotional and behavioral problems among parents, which could furthermore influence how they nurture and raise their children.

Future problems are described below. This research was unable to sufficiently study the adaptability of mothers and children in their new communities since April 2012, one year after the time of the earthquake. Evacuees live varied and diverse lives, and as the decision to return home becomes more difficult (Fukushima Minyū, 2014), the first issue that should be looked into in the future is what kind of interpersonal relationships evacuee families will build in accordance with the continuously changing conditions. Consequently, the second task should be to study what sort of long-term effects the experience of the earthquake disaster and the evacuation will have on the future lives of evacuee families. It seems that the evacuees themselves have been increasingly raising their own voices in regard to the transformation of their own philosophies on life since around 2013. That shows that this was a turning point (Sugiura, 2004) for the life of the evacuees of this disaster, and moreover, it seems to suggest that there is a need to understand the effects of the earthquake and the evacuation from a life-long development perspective.

Finally, this is something we have felt since we first interviewed the evacuee families, but when the evacuees spoke, we did not forget that there was a possibility that the evacuees were "performing" for the researchers by exaggerating the harshness and sadness of their situations as evacuees (in order to meet researchers' expectations). If researchers are unaware of this possibility, they will be unable to grasp the experiences and emotions of the evacuees, and they may paint a stereotypical picture of evacuees. We must take care to avoid this and continue to think about what we can do for evacuees who "simply want to live a normal life."

Acknowledgement

We would like to express our sincere appreciation to Family A, Family B and everyone at the Evacuee Families Group who showed great interest in this study and the support offered and took the time to cooperate. In addition, this project was only made possible through the cooperation of numerous current and former members of the Developmental Ethology Laboratory including undergraduate students. We would particularly like to express our thanks to Maiko Noda, Kanako Yonezawa, and Kimiyo Aikawa for putting us in contact with the evacuee families, providing assistance in analyzing the data, and so on.

References

Conger, R.d., Donnellan, M. B., 2007. An interactionist perspective on the socioeconomic context of human development. *Annual Review of Psychology*, 58, 175 – 199.

Fukushima Minyū shinbun, 2014. *Hinansha, nayami ōki seikatsu saiken, kaeru bekika... hinan saki ni nokoruka.* [Rebuilding lives for evacuees facing many troubles: Should they come home? Should they stay in their new communities?], Available from: http://www.minyu-net.com/osusume/daisinsai/serial/140911-2/news1.html, [Accessed 31 October 2014]

Hirata, S., Ishijima, K., Mochida, R., Shiraga, A., 2012. *Kasasagi purojekuto ni yoru shinsai hinan kazoku no shien.* [Support for families forced to live separately due to the Fukushima nuclear disaster: an interim report of the *Kasasagi* Project.], *Human Science Research*, 25 (2), 265-272.

Hirata, S., Ishijima, K., Mochida, R., Negayama, K., 2013. *Shinsai hinan kazoku no shien – kasasagi purojekuto no katsudō.* [Supporting families evacuating earthquakes: activities of the *Kasasagi* Project.], In: Tsujiuchi, T. (Ed.), *Gajyumaru teki shien no susume – hitori hitori no kokoro ni yorisou: higashi nihon daishinsai to ningen kagaku 1.* [The Great East Japan Earthquake and Human Science 1: Recommendations of Banyan-like Support – Getting closer to each individual.], Waseda University Booklet, After the Disaster 31, Waseda University Press, pp. 17-39.

Hosaka, Y., 2003. *Akushon risāchi.* [Action Research.], Muto, T., Yamada, Y., Minami, H., Sato, T., (Eds.), *Shitsuteki shinrigaku – sōzō teki ni katsuyō suru kotsu.* [Tips for creative qualitative psychology research.], Kitaōji Shobō.

Konno, Y., Sato, S., 2014. *Higashi nihon daishinsai oyobi genpatsu jiko ni yoru Fukushima kengai eno hinan no jittai (I) – boshi hinansha eno intabyū chōsa wo chūshin ni.* [Conditions surrounding evacuation from Fukushima Prefecture due to 2011 Tohoku Earthquake and nuclear power plant accident I: Focusing on interviews with mothers who evacuated with children.], *Memoirs of Faculty of Education and Human Studies, Akita University. Educational science*, 69, 145-157.

Negayama, K., Hirata, S., Ishijima, K., 2012. *Genpatsu jiko ni yoru hinan kazoku eno shien.* [Supporting families evacuating nuclear accidents.], *Practical Clinical Developmental Psychology Research*, 7, 42-46.

Reconstruction Agency, 2014. *Zenkoku no hinansha tō no kazu.* [Number of evacuees nationwide.], Available from: http://www.reconstruction.go.jp/topics/main-cat2/sub-cat2-1/20141031_hinansha.pdf, [Accessed 31 October 2014]

Sugiura, T., 2004. *Tenki no shinrigaku.* [The Psychology of Turning Points.], Nakanishiya Publishing.

Yamane, S., 2013. *Genpatsu jiko ni yoru "boshi hinan" mondai to sono shien – Yamagata-ken ni okeru hinansha chōsa dēta kara.* [Issues with "mother-child evacuation" after the nuclear accident and support – From data gathered from surveys of evacuees in Yamagata Prefecture.], *Yamagata University Faculty of Literature and Social Sciences Annual Report*, 10, 37-51.

8 Mental Health / Community Health / Environmental Health

Analysis of living conditions and intentions of out-of-prefecture evacuees fleeing the Fukushima nuclear power plant accident

Noriko Ishikawa MA[*1] *(Architectural Studies),*
Takaya Kojima PhD[*2][*3] *(Architectural Environmental Studies)*

Key words: Tohoku earthquake, Fukushima nuclear plant accident,
evaluating living environments, privately-rented temporary
housing, housing requisition system

I. Introduction

1. Research Goals

It has been four years since the accident at the Tokyo Electric Company Fukushima Daiichi Nuclear Power Plant that resulted from the 2011 Tohoku earthquake and tsunami disaster. However, many people who evacuated out of the prefecture are still forced to live in temporary housing. The requisitioning of residential space[1] for use as temporary emergency housing has been extended year by year and has now become a long-term fact of life. In addition, regarding the return of evacuees to their homes, while funding for requisitions for people moving to Fukushima from outside the prefecture has been approved, moves to locations outside of the prefecture are

---

*1 Graduate School of Human Sciences, Waseda University
*2 Professor, Faculty of Human Sciences, Waseda University
*3 Waseda Institute of Medical Anthropology on Disaster Reconstruction (WIMA)

---

1) Residential housing requisition system: This system is based on the flexible interpretation of Article 23, Paragraph 1, Item 1 (on the provision of accommodation facilities (i.e. emergency temporary housing)) of the Disaster Relief Act. In the case of a large-scale disaster, in order to quickly secure housing for victims of the disaster who lose their own homes, the Disaster Relief Act allows for prefectures accepting evacuees to requisition/lease private rental housing and offer such housing to evacuees.

218   Part II - 8

essentially unapproved, and must be paid by the individuals themselves. With no prospects in sight, out-of-prefecture evacuees are facing changing needs and being forced to make the difficult decision between laying down roots in the communities to which they have evacuated or returning to Fukushima.

With these facts in mind, this paper lays out the results of a mail-based survey designed to gain a better understanding of the living conditions and intentions of Fukushima residents living as evacuees in Saitama Prefecture and Tokyo Metropolis. Regarding analysis methodology, living environments were evaluated by comparing ownership rates and residence types before and after the disaster, and by comparing levels of satisfaction with living environments at points two and three years after the disaster. Evacuee intentions were investigated by targeting inhabitants of requisitioned housing, gaining an understanding of difference in intention as it related to rent payment method, and by looking into, comparing by age and family type, what sorts of factors influenced the intent to change living accommodations. Using the acquired knowledge of living environments and intentions, we then present recommendations on future issues that will be faced in rebuilding after large-scale disasters.

2. Summary of Survey

This analysis[2] is based on a mail survey sent to former Fukushima residents living in Saitama Prefecture and Tokyo Metropolis after having evacuated from Fukushima due to the 2011 Tohoku earthquake disaster and the subsequent nuclear power plant accident. The first survey was conducted between March and April 2013, two years after the disaster, with questionnaires sent to 4,268 evacuee households. The second survey was conducted between March and April 2014, with questionnaires sent to 3,599 evacuee households. A total of 530 responses were received for the 2013 survey (12.4% response rate), and 772 were received for the 2014 survey (21.5% response rate).

3. Number of out-of-prefecture evacuees, and number of moves made

According to Fukushima prefectural government reports, there were 47,149 out-of-prefecture evacuees living around the country as of March 2014, with 5,077 of those in Saitama Prefecture and 6,296 in Tokyo. As of the 2014 survey, the average number of moves made per household was 4.6 in Saitama and 4.3 in Tokyo, with the number of moves in the previous year standing at 0.6 for both Saitama and Tokyo. Hokugo et al (2006) conducted a survey in the disaster area after the 1995 Kobe Earthquake and

---

2) This paper is based on analysis of questionnaires conducted in March 2013 and March 2014 through the cooperation of the Shinsai Shien Network Saitama (SSN) and Waseda University's Disaster and Human Science Project.

reported that the average number of moves from evacuation center to temporary housing to rebuilt public housing was 3.05. Considering that former Fukushima's households are still currently evacuated outside of the prefecture, we can say that they will have made two or three moves more than the number of moves mentioned in the survey of the Kobe Earthquake.

II. Change related to dissatisfaction with living environment before and after disaster

1. Change in living conditions before and after disaster

Home ownership in Fukushima before the disaster stood at 80% with almost 90% being houses. The 2014 survey conducted three years after the disaster found that the majority of evacuee households were renting (62.0% in Saitama and 57.6% in Tokyo), and the majority of homes were in multi-unit buildings (62.8% in Saitama, 81.4% in Tokyo). (See Table 1.)

Comparing the surveys, we learn that current 2014 home ownership rates increased in both Saitama and Tokyo over the 2013 survey, and the number of households renting is trending downwards. Regarding residence type, there was also an increase in numbers of those living in houses between 2013 and 2014 in both Saitama and Tokyo, and the number of evacuees living in multi-unit housing is also trending downwards. Comparing by region, there was a larger change in ownership and residence type for those in Saitama than those in Tokyo. These responses show that, as of three years after the disaster, there was a certain number of households that had already purchased houses in areas to which they had evacuated, and that those numbers were increasing.

Table 1. Annual change in home ownership rates and residence type (Units: %)

		Fukushima Prefecture Pre-disaster	Saitama Prefecture		Tokyo Metropolis	
			2013	2014	2013	2014
Ownership	Owned	80.1	9.4	17.1	5.8	10.3
	Rented	12.7	72.8	62.0	61.9	57.6
	Company housing	1.9	2.8	2.7	8.1	2.7
	Lodger	0.9	2.4	5.6	5.4	8.4
	Evacuation center	—	4.7	—	3.1	—
	Other	4.0	7.1	10.7	15.7	19.7
	No response	0.4	0.8	1.9	0.0	1.4
Residence Type	House	88.5	24.3	30.2	10.0	12.4
	Multi-unit	9.8	72.4	62.8	89.5	81.4
	Other	0.5	3.3	5.6	0.5	4.9
	No response	1.2	4.5	1.3	1.8	1.4

2. Overall evaluation of residence and residential surroundings

In order to compare living environment evaluations with the general public, reference was made to the evaluation items in the "2008 Comprehensive Lifestyle Survey" conducted by the Ministry of Land, Infrastructure, Transport and Tourism (MLIT). The following question was posed: "How do you feel overall about your current residence and the surrounding area?" Respondents were asked to answer on a scale of 1 to 4, from "very satisfied" to "very dissatisfied." National, Kanto, and Tohoku dissatisfaction rates (somewhat and very dissatisfied) for each item were taken from the 2008 Comprehensive Lifestyle Survey and are presented in Figure 1 alongside the annual dissatisfaction rates for Saitama and Tokyo as determined by this survey.

No major changes were seen in total dissatisfaction rates for residence plus residential surroundings in Saitama, which rose only slightly between 2013 and 2014 to 41.2%, but rates in Tokyo rose 4.9 points from 2013 to 2014 to 38.1%. Residence dissatisfaction dropped 4.9 points in Saitama between 2013 and 2014 to 54.5%, and rose 8.1 points to 54.3% in Tokyo in the same period. Comparing regional numbers, we find that dissatisfaction rates in Saitama were higher than in Tokyo for all items surveyed.

Comparing to the National, Kanto, and Tohoku numbers in the Comprehensive Lifestyle Survey aimed at the general public, residence dissatisfaction in this survey was higher in both Saitama and Tokyo, but dissatisfaction in residential surroundings was lower for Tokyo. In other words, evacuees to Tokyo clearly tend to be more satisfied with their residential surroundings than members of the general public.

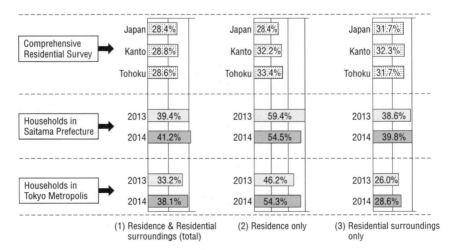

Figure 1. Residence and residential surroundings dissatisfaction rates

3. Itemized evaluation of residence and residential surroundings in evacuation destinations

To gain a better understanding of the composition of evacuee living environment evaluations, factor analysis (maximum-likelihood estimation, promax rotational solution) was conducted using evaluations made on the same 1 to 4 satisfaction scale described above in Section 2 pertaining to 12 items dealing with residence and 10 items dealing with residential surroundings surveyed in 2014. Factor analysis is used to find common factors that aid in summarizing the reasons behind why certain answers were provided. Figure 2 presents dissatisfaction rates (somewhat + very dissatisfied) by year (2013 and 2014) and region (Saitama Prefecture and Tokyo Metropolis) based on the results of the factor analysis and sorted by evaluation item. In order to compare to members of the general public, the national results from the Comprehensive Lifestyle Survey are also included. Derived factors for residence were interpreted as "F1: residence function" and "F2: Size", while factors for residential surroundings were interpreted as "F1: Safety/security" and "F2: Convenience."

Neither Saitama nor Tokyo saw major changes in the dissatisfaction rates for each item between 2013 and 2014. When comparing by region (Saitama, Tokyo) residence function (F1) dissatisfaction rate was higher in Saitama. Dissatisfaction rates for items related to residential surroundings safety/security (F1) was also higher in Saitama. Comparing to the national numbers in the Comprehensive Lifestyle Survey, we find that the rate of dissatisfaction with regard to residence size (F2) remain extremely

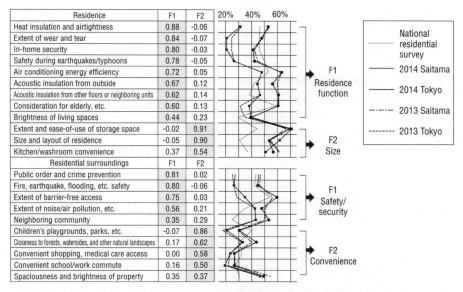

Figure 2. Factor analysis and dissatisfaction rate of residence and residential surroundings

222   Part II - 8

high. In addition, there is little difference seen in dissatisfaction rates regarding convenience when compared to the general public.

4. Issues with residence size in evacuation destinations

Given the above-mentioned high dissatisfaction rates regarding size, in order to clarify how much living area is needed in a home, we made use of the minimum living area standard[3] (MLAS) calculation method recommended by MLIT to judge between pre-disaster MLAS and MLAS in current residences. Moreover, 53.8% of households in Saitama and 56% of those in Tokyo saw changes in the number of people living in each household from before the disaster, so we also present the ratios for those under the MLAS as calculated using the number of individuals in each household before the disaster (Fig. 3). The percentage of evacuees living in residences not meeting MLAS values is 14% in Saitama, a four-point drop from 2013, and 15.9% in Tokyo, a ten-point drop from 2013. Calculating the same numbers using the pre-disaster household size, we find that 22.1% of households in Saitama and 26.5% of households in Tokyo would be below the MLAS. According to a 2008 survey conducted by the Ministry of Internal Affairs and Communications Statistics Bureau, the number of households under the MLAS was 5% for Fukushima, 9% for Saitama, and 21% for Tokyo. This illustrates that most evacuees had been living in homes of satisfactory size in Fukushima before the disaster. However, the size of the homes in which the evacuees currently live is lower than the MLAS for a certain number of households, and some wrote that they are dissatisfied with the amount of space they have whenever their scattered family gathers and because their children are growing. In addition, 21% of respondents answered that they "have no space to gather the family in one place" as "a reason for why they are unable to spend time with family members living in the same home."

5. Evaluation of Fukushima residence and current residence

As previously mentioned, most evacuees owned detached houses in Fukushima before the disaster, but after the disaster, 80% of evacuees moved into multi-unit residential housing. When choosing to leave the prefecture, it is obvious that they did not have the leeway to carefully scrutinize their new living environments with consideration given to the prospect of living there long term. Ishikawa and Kojima (2014) conducted a covariance structure analysis on living environment evaluation pre- and post-disaster, and the results showed that a comparative evaluation with the former residence in Fukushima had an influence on the evaluation of layout and space in the

---

3) Minimum living area standard (MLAS) calculated by MLIT: the living area standard as laid out in the Basic Housing Plan. Calculated by number of individuals in a household, and considered to be the minimum area necessary to live a healthy and culturally-rich lifestyle. Single-person household: 25 m², two-person household: 30 m², three-person household: 40 m².

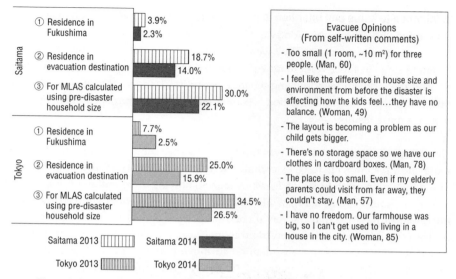

Figure 3. Percentage of households in residences below minimum living area standard

evacuation destination residence. The analysis suggested that one factor behind the drop in living space in Tokyo were an average income under 4,000,000 yen and evacuation from areas issued with lower-urgency evacuation orders. In other words, it is possible that there was an economic effect caused by the differences in compensation awarded in line with evacuation order urgency. Under the housing requisition system, rent is set at under 75,000 yen (under 100,000 yen for five or more inhabitants). Convenience and size are reflected in rental fees, so it is possible that differences in economic concerns had an influence on residence selection.

III. Intention to settle and intention to move among out-of-prefecture evacuees

1. Current situation regarding inhabitants of requisitioned housing

A 2008 report by the Tokyo Metropolitan Government Bureau of General Affairs stated that, in regard to future expectations of Tokyo and prefectures of birth, a majority wished for housing support (827 responses or 54%), followed by health and welfare support (661 responses or 44%). In our 2014 survey, the largest proportion of evacuees were renting residences under the housing requisition system in both Saitama and Tokyo. In Saitama, the number was 44.1%, a 5.5-point drop from 2013, and in Tokyo the number was 30.5%, a drop of 3.6 points since 2013. In addition, while the housing requisition system is being extended annually, the number of respondents who answered that they "feel the system has issues" was 51% in Saitama and 63% in Tokyo.

2. Intention to settle and intention to move in residents of requisitioned housing

Users of the housing requisition system were asked, "Do you want to continue living in your current residence?" They were asked to select responses ranging from 1 for "want to stay" to 4 for "want to move", considering three potential changes in conditions: if the requisitioned housing tenancy period is extended; if rent is set at a low rate; and if the residential situation is converted to a regular rental contract. Figure 4 displays these results.

No annual change of intention was found in either Saitama or Tokyo if the housing requisition system were to be extended. There was a difference in result for this condition by region, with 61.1% of Tokyo evacuees showing an intention to settle (want to stay + would rather stay), while 41.7% of Saitama evacuees showed the same intention. In the case that the rental conditions were converted to a regular rental contract (with fees), Saitama showed no change year-on-year, while the percentage of Tokyo residents expressing an intention to move (want to move + would rather move) rose 11.2 points to 58.0% from 2013 to 2014. A difference was seen regarding intention to settle in the 2014 survey in the case that rent was set at a low rate, with Saitama at 22.8% and 47.7% for Tokyo. In other words, if a low rent began to be charged, the proportion of Saitama evacuees intending to move was high, while the proportion of Tokyo evacuees intending to stay was high.

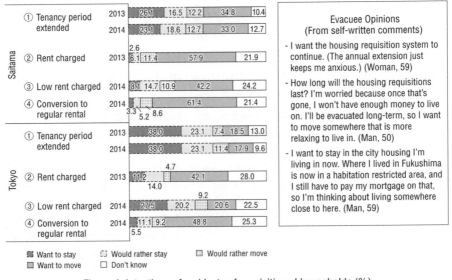

Figure 4. Intentions of residents of requisitioned households (%)

Ishikawa, Tsujiuchi, Masuda, and Kojima (2014) investigated what living environment evaluation items were factors in influencing users of the housing requisition system to want to stay in their current residence by conducting a multiple population simultaneous covariance structure analysis for Saitama and Tokyo (Fig. 5). That analysis found that in both Saitama and Tokyo, residence size and neighboring community greatly influenced the latent variable: evacuee intention to stay in their current residence. In addition, the results suggested that intention to stay for Tokyo evacuees was directly influenced by convenience of their work/school commute.

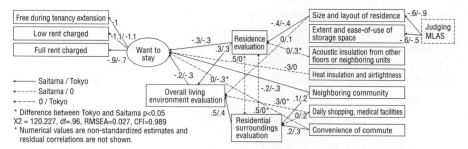

Figure 5. Intention model for residents in requisitioned housing (2014 survey)

3. Intention to move by age group

Correspondence analysis was conducted on all respondents to the 2014 survey in order to clarify the basic axes on which objectives behind intentions to move could be placed (Fig. 6). Attributes utilized were age (20 to 80 years), sex, region (Saitama/Tokyo), change in household size, the 26 items of intention objectives, desired place to live (in six levels from current location to home in Fukushima), and level of worry about radiation exposure (ra 1 to 10). Furthermore, each intention objective corresponds to a response that combines the first and second selections. Correspondence analysis is a method used to position measurement items and subjects in the same space, and items/subjects with a highly corresponding relationship will appear close to each other when plotted.

Analysis results revealed two main axes, the first axis (vertical) and second axis (horizontal). The vertical axis (contribution rate 49%) fell in line with age group, and was interpreted as being the axis determining desire to return to Fukushima (negative direction) and impossibility to return Fukushima (positive direction). On the other hand, the horizontal axis (contribution rate 16%) shows intention decisions regarding residence followed a trend of emphasizing comfort (negative direction) and emphasizing safety and security (positive direction). Reviewing each of the elements plotted on these two axes allowed for the interpretation that each element was roughly separated by age along the vertical axis. Characteristics of each age group are presented in Table 2, and main intention objectives by age group are presented in Figure 7 in the order of value on axis 1, the component clarified by the correspondence analysis. These results showed that the child-raising age group is largely worried about radiation exposure and emphasized a child-rearing environment in their selection not to return to Fukushima. The elderly age group was less worried about radiation exposure and placed more priority on nursing care and other daily living issues, and a high proportion expressed a desire to return to Fukushima. Iwai (2014) also conducted a survey that, like this paper, found that regardless of the proportion of the population of areas in Fukushima that are difficult to return to, the younger the household, the more likely they were to respond that they had already "decided not to return." As the comments showed, many truly want to return if they could lead the same life they led before the disaster. However, currently many seem to be forced to select the responses, "want to go back but can't" or "don't want to go back but have no choice."

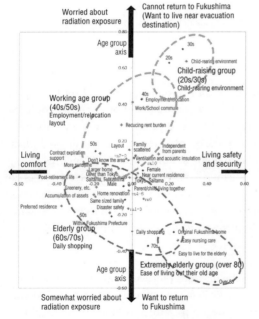

Figure 6. Correspondence analysis on intention to move

Table 2. Characteristics of each age group

Child-raising age (20s-30s)	This age group places an emphasis on child-rearing environment, is greatly concerned about radiation exposure, and wants to stay close to current residence in evacuation destination or move somewhere else in Saitama/Tokyo.
Working age (40s-50s)	The intention of a high proportion is based upon objectives centered on work, i.e. commuting/relocating, living with other family members, and wanting a new home layout. Greatly concerned about radiation exposure, a large proportion have chosen not to return to Fukushima.
Elderly (60s-70s)	This group puts emphasis on improving access to daily shopping, medical care, and other items of convenience. Levels of worry about radiation exposure are varied, as are the areas to which this group wants to move.
Extremely elderly (80s)	Prioritizes ease-of-life for elderly individuals, nursing care, and other objectives. Tendency towards lower levels of concern about radiation exposure, and a large proportion wants to return to Fukushima.

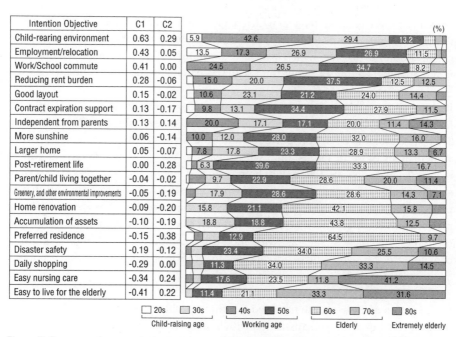

Figure 7. Correspondence analysis components regarding intention objectives and proportions by age group

IV. Issues facing long-term out-of-prefecture evacuees in rebuilding their lives

The 2011 Tohoku Earthquake worsened with the Fukushima nuclear power plant accident and resulted individuals evacuating outside of the prefecture – a large difference from previous natural disaster. Three years since the disaster, we find that its victims are facing considerable difficulties in adapting to their new living environments. The survey of living environment evaluations and future intentions conducted with out-of-prefecture evacuees illustrates a number of issues that will be faced in rebuilding after future large-scale disasters, and provides for some recommendations.

1. Evaluating living environments

Dissatisfaction with residences in evacuation destinations continues. Around 50% of families have been separated, resulting in dissatisfaction regarding people's inability to gather widely-flung family members in one place, and dissatisfaction with the amount of space children have in which to grow. As the evacuation is prolonged, it is thought that this will result in people ending up with a poor balance between communication and privacy, which will have an influence on their relationships with family members living elsewhere and with those living in the same residence.

In the evaluation of convenience, etc. of residential surroundings, there was little difference seen between the responses of evacuees and those of the general public. Both Tokyo and Saitama have transportation and other things considered to be more convenient than those in Fukushima, which leads to the good evaluation for convenience. There is dissatisfaction with home size and layout, but 40% of evacuees were satisfied with convenient commutes to work and school. From this we find that in people's decisions to remain in the evacuation destination, there was less of a priority placed on living space in the home, and more on meeting up with distant family, and on living conveniences such as work and school commutes. In addition, regarding convenience and size, as these are reflected in rental fees, it is possible that economic concerns had an influence on residence selection.

Prolongation of the evacuation has led to various problems, such as households moving four times or more, dissatisfaction with living arrangements, and family relationships suffering. If this situation is expected to continue, it will become necessary to review the duration of the Disaster Relief Act, and to consider implementation of policies within the current housing requisition system to include standards for household numbers and rental amounts, and to allow for the selection of residential layouts/sizes that take into account dispersal of family members, age of children, etc.

2. Intentions of out-of-prefecture evacuees

It was found that intentions regarding settling and/or moving among users of the housing requisition system were dependent on the means of rental payments. In addition, levels of concern about radiation exposure and intention objectives differed by age group with a clear distinction in that younger evacuees want to stay in the evacuation destination, and the desire to return to Fukushima increased with an increase in group age.

The housing requisition system has been extended annually and is set to be in place until March 2016. However, while households are approved to take advantage of the system when returning to Fukushima Prefecture, out-of-prefecture moves are essentially not approved. Considering the prolonged nature of the situation, and assuming the major premises of securing employment and income, there needs to be consideration given to individual circumstances, including an environment for children, worries about radiation exposure, and conveniences needed for life.

One future task will be to review measures that would allow people to select between "stable settlement" and "move to a new home" – such measures would be useful in providing out-of-prefecture evacuees with prospects for the future that are in accordance with their own needs.

Note: This report is a reorganization of the information presented in Ishikawa and Kojima (2014) and Ishikawa, Tsujiuchi, Masuda, and Kojima (2014) with additional analysis and discussion.

Acknowledgements

This research was made possible through the cooperation of the Shinsai Shien Network Saitama (represented by Tadashi Inomata) and the Waseda University Disaster and Human Science Project (represented by Takuya Tsujiuchi and Kazutaka Masuda). We would like to express our gratitude to all victims who responded to the questionnaire survey and to everyone concerned.

In addition, this research was supported by the MEXT Programme for Strategic Research Base Foundation Support Projects at Private Universities (represented by Hiroaki Kumano, the 2012 Fukushima Prefectural Comprehensive Regional Planning Support Program (support for maintaining and rehabilitating hometowns and connections) Subsidies, and the 2013 Welfare and Medical Service Agency Social Welfare Promotion Subsidies Program.

References

Disaster Recovery Support Division, Bureau of General Affairs, Tokyo Metropolitan Government, 2013. *Tonai hinan sha ankēto chōsa kekka.* [Results of questionnaire survey of evacuees in Tokyo.]

Fukushima Prefectural Evacuee Support Section. Available from: http://www.pref. fukushima.lg.jp/sec/16055b/ [Accessed 17 December 2018]

Hokugo, A., Higuchi, D., Murosaki Y., 2006. *Hanshin Awaji dai shinsai kara mita jyūtaku saiken shien no arikata.* [Supporting housing reconstruction from the perspectives of the Kobe Earthquake.], *Urban Housing Sciences,* 53, 86 -97.

Housing Policy Division, Housing Bureau, Ministry of Land, Infrastructure, Transport and Tourism. *Heisei 20 nen jyūtaku sōgō chōsa.* [2008 Comprehensive Lifestyle Survey.], e-Stat official government statistics portal, Available from: http://www.mlit.go.jp/report/press/house02_hh_000035.html [Accessed 17 December 2018]

Ishikawa, N., Kojima, T., 2014. *Fukushima genpatsu jiko ni yoru kengai hinan sha no jūkankyo hyōka ni kansuru kenkyū – Tōkyō-to to Saitama-ken wo bunseki taishō ni shite.* [A study on living environment evaluation by out-of-prefecture Fukushima nuclear power plant accident evacuees: Analysis of Tokyo Metropolis and Saitama Prefecture.], Summaries of Technical Papers of Annual Meeting, D1, Architectural Institute of Japan, pp. 55-56.

Ishikawa, N., Tsujiuchi, T., Masuda, K., Kojima, T., 2014. *Fukushima genpatsu jiko ni yoru kengai hinan sha no jūkankyo ni kansuru kenkyū.* [A study on living environments of out-of-prefecture Fukushima nuclear power plant evacuees.], The Behaviormetric Society 42nd Conference Presentation Paper Proceedings, pp. 244.

Iwai, N., 2014. *Genpatsu hinan ni kansuru jyūmin ikō chōsa – shakai chōsa no shiten kara mita kadai.* [Surveys on Life Conditions and Future Prospects of Nuclear Accident Evacuees: Points to be examined from a perspective of social survey methodology.], *Trends in the Sciences,* 94-101.

Statistics Bureau, Ministry of Internal Affairs and Communications, 2008. *Jyūtaku, tochi tōkei chōsa, Heisei 20 nendo ban.* [Housing/land statistical survey 2008.], Available from: http://www.stat.go.jp/data/jyutaku/2008/nihon/5_2.htm [Accessed 17 December 2018]

9 Community Health / Policy Making / Social Security

Compensation for damages caused by the nuclear power plant disaster

Hiroshi Kitamura[1][2] *(Political Science)*

Key words: compensation, nuclear power plant disaster, Tokyo Electric Power Company (TEPCO), national policy, responsibilities

I. Introduction

The accident at the Fukushima Daiichi Nuclear Power Plant caused tremendous damage. The prospect for a resolution to the situation is currently still slim, as damage is still being caused by harmful rumors and other means, and an accurate assessment of the situation cannot be obtained. Contamination by radiation is widespread and the region eligible for compensation is expanding to a considerably larger area. As the region expands geographically, the seriousness of the situation is increasing. A lot of people forced to evacuate from homes that stood within the designated evacuation zone face particularly difficult hardships.

Many of the residents living within 20 km of the nuclear plant found themselves being moved to distant places, with the local government bodies also being forced to relocate to continue offering services. Even areas greater than 20 km from the nuclear plant were required to evacuate depending on radiation levels, and there were evacuees from other regions who voluntarily evacuated.

Evacuees ended up scattered across the country, mainly within Fukushima, but many found themselves evacuated to such places in the capital region as Tokyo and Saitama, Niigata, and so on. Conditions surrounding the evacuation were particularly urgent immediately after the accident and were just the same as an great escape,

---

[1] Senior Researcher, Institute of Politics and Economy
[2] Visiting Researcher, Waseda Institute of Medical Anthropology on Disaster Reconstruction (WIMA)

an exodus. It gradually became clear that people would not be able to return home soon, and the evacuation essentially turned into diaspora. In that sense, it became possible to look at the evacuees as internally-displaced persons and examine the situation as a refugee issue.

II. The damage compensation framework and the current situation

According to nuclear disaster law as laid out in the "Act on Compensation for Nuclear Damage," the framework for compensating for damage caused by a nuclear accident makes the party involved in an accident, in this case Tokyo Electric Power Company (TEPCO), assume unlimited responsibility. Although, as the amount of compensation TEPCO can provide is limited, it was ultimately decided that the nation/government would provide compensation.

This type of situation wasn't anticipated in the original law, and it wasn't clear what form compensation would take, so the Nuclear Damage Compensation Facilitation Corporation Act was enacted to lay out such a framework. However, rather than force TEPCO to take suitable responsibility, this act prioritized saving the company, and was essentially designed to maintain the existing power supply system.

That is how the compensation process was begun without providing the opportunity to fundamentally reflect upon the inherent issues with nuclear power generation, which had, in a manner of speaking, been promoted as national policy. TEPCO showed little awareness of it having been at the nucleus of the accident, and it would be difficult to say that it showed sufficient awareness of its responsibility for it. As would be expected, the government expected TEPCO to provide damage compensation, but in fact, seemed rather to be aiming to ensure TEPCO's survival, and it continued to lean towards maintaining nuclear power production without implementing sufficient changes to energy policy.

There were many problems inherent to that situation including the dishonest and trivialized explanations given regarding the actual extent of the damage caused from the beginning of the accident.

Here I would like to provide a simple explanation of compensation procedures and flow thus far.

1. Temporary payments of damage compensation
TEPCO is providing guaranteed temporary payments mainly to residents of the designated evacuation zones who lost the foundations upon which their lives were built.

Compensation for damages caused by the nuclear power plant disaster   233

Specific amounts have already been paid, and the payments are designed as a temporary source of funding which has to be paid promptly.

Claims are based on damage estimates and can be paid off upon confirmation of the amount of damage done, but if temporary payments are seen as temporary sources of funding, problems arise with regards to donations. Issues may also arise between the parties involved.

2. Dispute Reconciliation Committee for Nuclear Damage Compensation

This government body was founded through the Act on Compensation for Nuclear Damage, and through the formulation of criteria for compensation from damage caused by the accident/disaster, it released interim guidelines in August, 2011 following the first and second guidelines in order to move the compensation process forward. TEPCO provides compensation in line with these criteria.

In addition, the Nuclear Damage Compensation Facilitation Corporation Act was enacted at the same time, and with it, the Nuclear Damage Compensation Facilitation Corporation was established. This corporation, through funding provided by the government, provides TEPCO with the financial support it needs to pay compensation. This strengthens the original, insufficient compensation payment scheme, and makes it more practical.

However, these interim guidelines still have inadequacies, and it has been pointed out that there are issues and problems that need to be resolved. The basis on which consolation payments for psychological trauma are calculated, and the amounts paid, have been criticized for not being enough, and it is possible that this will become a future point of contention. The largest unresolved issue is the response to those residents of the area up to 30 km from the power plant who elected to undergo voluntary evacuation. Additional guidelines must be designed to resolve these issues continue to be released, and the debate regarding those guidelines continues to grow.

3. Nuclear Damage Compensation Dispute Resolution Center

The Nuclear Damage Compensation Dispute Resolution Center was established as an arbitration body for the compensation claims and it is positioned to serve as an Alternative Dispute Resolution (ADR) organization. During the arbitration process, once an application is received, arbiters comprised of lawyers and the like for both parties confirm the facts of the case, and a mediation plan is presented. The claim ends there if that plan resolves the issues, but if not, the case must go to court. The number of cases is expected to grow vastly, and court cases take time, so the center became necessary in order to provide prompter responses.

Dispute Resolution Centers have currently been established in two locations – in Tokyo and Koriyama, Fukushima – and applications are already being accepted. At this point, the problems surrounding consolation payments for psychological trauma are major points of contention, but it is expected that the response to voluntary evacuees will become a major focus in the future.

4. The formation of legal relief teams and support organizations

The text above provides a rough idea of the framework and flow for providing damage compensation. TEPCO pays compensation based on the guidelines laid out by the Dispute Reconciliation Committee for Nuclear Damage Compensation. If an agreement cannot be reached there, arbitration is provided through the nuclear damage compensation ADR process, and if no resolution is found there, a lawsuit is filed, and the case goes to trial in the end.

Presently, there are several movements of lawyers providing support for damage compensation claims. The damage caused by the nuclear disaster, which includes damage from harmful rumors, has affected a wide range of people, spreading as far as the agriculture and fishing industries, and the response must be as diverse as the range of victims.

As the damage caused by rumors must also be included, areas have been affected to an extent that exceeds the damage caused directly by the accident. In addition, when providing compensation, it is difficult to calculate the costs incurred by people when they are forced to evacuate. Even when the extent and the timing of the damage can be confirmed, claimants must provide their own proof, which is difficult to do when damage is still being caused. In order to calculate damages, claimants must individually gather their own proof (e.g. receipts showing costs incurred during the evacuation) and submit it themselves.

When damage still continues to be suffered, claims are separated into time periods, and claimants can apply for compensation in multiple stages. Nevertheless this is difficult, as individual, concrete evidence must be provided by the claimant.

In particular, claims submitted to TEPCO were initially very complicated and could not be filled out easily. On top of that, applicants were asked to agree not to file any objections after a claim had been filed. TEPCO faced a large amount of criticism because its attitude was far from that of a company that was aiming sincerely to provide compensation for damages. This behavior on the part of TEPCO made people suspicious that the company was hoping that most victims would abandon their claims due to the difficulty of the process.

Compensation for damages caused by the nuclear power plant disaster   235

In response to this situation, bar associations in Fukushima (and in Tokyo, Saitama and other prefectures where many evacuees were living) began to hold meetings to explain the system of compensation for damage caused by the nuclear accident. To help attendees prepare their damage compensation claims, for example, they were provided with nuclear disaster damage notebooks and other items they could use to collect evidence for their claims and record future health issues.

As concrete claim procedures were developed, and to a certain extent, when the bar associations began holding explanatory meetings on damage compensation, legal experts in various areas began voluntarily setting up nuclear disaster relief legal teams. Currently, such teams work in Tokyo, Saitama and other areas, and they are now active in Fukushima with the support of lawyers from various areas.

Through ADR conflict mediation, lawsuits and other means, victims will receive relief for the damage they suffer, but depending on the case, group litigation and applications may be reviewed, and they are expected to grow considerably.

In addition, specific support organizations lie behind the formation of the legal teams in Tokyo, Saitama and other areas where the movements began comparatively quickly. Naturally, prompt responses on the part of the bar associations also played a large role, but in these areas, lawyers were already leading victim support efforts, and they were able to harness those experiences.

The work of the Japanese Federation of Bar Associations (JFBA) should also be noted. The JFBA criticized TEPCO's behavior regarding compensation claim procedures and other issues, and also actively made recommendations in regard to the compensation framework itself. Regarding compensation, the JFBA called for a cautious response towards the claim documents provided by TEPCO and provided pamphlets that presented the possibility of having damage compensation processed through ADR and multiple alternative methods.

III. Recommendations and arguments to be considered

The nuclear accident and scale of the damage caused by the accident were considerable, and similar to previous large-scale disasters, a large number of issues related to damage compensation have appeared. It is necessary to review these issues and consider how compensation will be provided in the future.

What must first be confirmed is where the final responsibility for the accident lies. In this case, Tokyo Electric Power Company was of course managing the production of electricity at the nuclear power plant, which means that the primary responsibility unmistakably lies with TEPCO. Therefore, TEPCO is the main party responsible for providing compensation/reparations, and the actual compensation process is being moved forward in line with this. Currently, the immense scale of the accident has resulted in TEPCO being unable to cover the entire amount, so the government has assumed responsibility for any amounts that exceed TEPCO's ability to pay.

The current supporting law was considered within this sort of framework, and though it is insufficient, up to this point the compensation system for nuclear disasters has been fundamentally based on such a position. In other words, responsibility essentially lies with operators. Direct responsibility is assigned in that way.

However, what level of responsibility should the government have? Can it be limited to assuming the financial burden that goes beyond TEPCO's ability to pay, or should the government also take responsibility for having promoted the nuclear power generation national policy that is now under such strict scrutiny? These questions must be answered when reviewing damage compensation and designing the system for providing it.

In previous cases of environmental pollution and other accidents, even when the operator assumed direct responsibility, legislation and other means were used to create a framework through which the government could provide compensation that went beyond the limits of the operator to pay. In contrast, the government did not clearly admit to any responsibility for damage caused by war or other events. However, in both cases, social movements seeking responsibility and compensation have caused the process to become a matter of dispute.

Let us now take a brief look at a few issues concerning compensation claims for damage caused by the nuclear accident, and at some specific recommendations.

1. The concept of responsibility

Examination of the basis of compensation for damage caused by the nuclear disaster has mainly been conducted from a legal perspective. However, it is necessary to consider the responsibility for the accident by taking a broader view. Considering the significance of the accident, even though it is natural to pursue legal responsibility, efforts must not stop there – questions regarding ethical and moral responsibility must also be answered. That allows for important suggestions to be provided from a different perspective even for damage compensation claims being moved forward within the legal framework.

The subjects of damage compensation claims lie within the scope of what can actually be proven. This basically amounts to the items that can be understood in a quan-

Compensation for damages caused by the nuclear power plant disaster   237

titative way, and for which calculation is possible. However, many victims, including those forced to evacuate from their homes, had the foundation of their lives completely undermined, and in such cases, the ethical and moral perspectives also require the formulation of a compensation scheme different from any previous scheme. It is not enough to consider the issue simply in terms of compensating for lost income.

One unique characteristic of this disaster is that victims were deprived of the foundation on which their lives were built, and subsequently, it became difficult for them to hold any hope for the future. It is difficult to gain a quantitative understanding of compensation that suits such conditions, and there are limits to how accurately a numerical value can be assigned. This differs somewhat from the consolation payments for psychological trauma. While it is similar in that psychological trauma is also difficult to quantify, we are discussing the loss of the foundations of a victim's entire life, so must we not also consider the compensation required to substitute for that foundations or rebuild that life?

In order for people to be able to live independently, TEPCO must support the victims every day until they achieve a certain level of lifestyle. This concept urges us to go beyond the legal perspective of responsibility and think more analytically.

The idea of more comprehensive compensation has been raised in previous cases involving the laying of responsibility for harm caused by environmental pollution, pharmaceutical drugs, and war and post-war events, and alongside the question of legal responsibility, raising issues socially has caused the idea to become a matter of dispute. Keeping in mind the differences between this and consolation payments, we can look at TEPCO's moral responsibility and recognize that this accident destroyed the lives, plans, and futures of many people. TEPCO should apologize for this and provide compensation and support to the victims.

However, TEPCO's actual attitude is far removed from such ideas. As with past experiences, people must raise the social issues and start social movements. It is necessary to do so using legal means to the greatest extent possible and use every possible method to determine where responsibility lies.

2. The significance of the nuclear accident and disaster
In order to clearly determine responsibility for this accident and the subsequent damages caused, it is necessary to consider its significance from a broader scope. The generation of power by nuclear means was made a part of national policy, but it also served as a symbol of modern science and technology. Reviewing this idea is needed, and it means a review of modernity. The compensation framework also brings with it

issues of where ethical responsibility lies, and changes in how compensation is paid. This process will help clarify the responsibility of the state/government.

National policy does not only refer to projects promoted by the government, even when the operator is a separate entity; it is also related to how society should be, as is indicated by the fact that energy policy itself is under review. From that perspective, it is necessary to clarify and discuss where the government's responsibility lies.

This includes a guarantee of safety made to citizens by the government and other public agencies – a guarantee that extends beyond reparation and compensation for damages, or the provision of compensation and support towards establishing a new life. By organizing our ideas around these concepts, we become able to also consider the ideological implications of the accident.

3. Regarding compensation for damages

This section points out a few specific issues connected to specific procedures for damage compensation.

First, TEPCO's attitude is a major problem, and judgements made by the nuclear plant ADR are very important. Even considering the premise that the ADR body is meant to pass down judgements from a neutral position, judgements made here will determine whether future resolution processes also proceed smoothly. Although lawsuits are currently unavoidable, determining compensation takes time, and judgements made through the ADR process are key to ensuring prompt responses. Thus, fair and reasonable results are needed.

Second, TEPCO's half-hearted attitude raises the possibility of people not receiving sufficient compensation if the situation remains the same, and it will become necessary for claimants to proceed collectively to ADR and lawsuits. Because of issues surrounding the calculation of compensation amounts, direct claims made through TEPCO are not going smoothly. For this reason, it is expected that collective action made with legal counsel from various areas and other types of support will be necessary to restore and assert the rights of claimants. The dispute resolution process is also taking on a collective form dependent on interests, regions, and issues. It is thought that the scale will become considerably large in some cases.

Third, even if there are problems with the damage compensation scheme, compensation should be immediately paid wherever possible, regardless of the form resolution takes and the time required. Where there is no room to contest a claim, payments must be made as soon as possible for compensation amounts already confirmed.

Fourth, the role of legal counsel is of course crucial, but volunteer support from the civil sector is also important. The compensation claims process is expected to be prolonged, and there is a large role for individual supporters and organizations to play. The accident must be seen as a society-wide issue, and it is necessary for efforts to be put into voluntary initiatives. This is also necessary in regard to clarifying the responsibilities of both TEPCO and the government for the purpose of asserting rights and realizing claims. In order to bring up these issues on a societal level, large-scale movements are particularly needed, and one important issue is how to build such movements.

Up until this point, victim support in the form of living and legal consultation has been a civil initiative lead by legal experts. It cannot be denied that this has had an influence on compensation issues, including from the social movement aspect. In the future, it will be necessary to clarify where responsibility lies and establish an argument regarding the right to make claims for compensation, and this will require scientific knowledge upon which to base the requisite theories.

However, it is possible that some tension will arise between the issues of victim support and the raising of societal level problems to ensuring damage compensation is paid. Although such movements are indispensable to the claiming of rights, they are fundamentally different from support. Although it is possible to start a movement for the empowerment of the victims, it should not be isolated from the parties involved and become a purpose.

Fifth, it is expected that, ultimately, new legislation will be required to come up with a resolution. Various issues and arguments will be brought to light during the claim process, and in the future, new laws will be needed to relieve the victims and resolve those issues.

The legal support structure consisting in the existing damage compensation framework is insufficient. It essentially is aimed at ensuring the survival of TEPCO and does not ensure sufficient assumption of responsibility on the part of TEPCO or the government. A more comprehensive compensation scheme is needed, as are policies to build it. Moreover, potential future issues could include a review of the existing electric power structure, and consideration of the possibility of splitting up power generation and transmission operations, or the liberalization of other areas of the electric power generation industry.

4. Other methods of making sure responsibilities are met

It is necessary to utilize as many methods as possible to make TEPCO fulfill its responsibilities. Various issues must be raised in regard to damage compensation claims, but we must also consider actions not directly related to compensation. Filing a shareholder lawsuit is one such option.

It is also necessary to continue asking about the cost of safety and the obligation to consider the safety of the people. The lawsuits filed to stop the operation of nuclear power plants are one way to force TEPCO to take responsibility, and will force discussion on the pros and cons of nuclear power.

TEPCO is not the only company operating nuclear power plants, and injunctions are being filed against other electric power companies to lead people to question the nuclear power development system itself. This is truly about raising issues and objecting to national policy, and it is important in the sense not only that it seeks for responsibilities to be filled, but also that it clarifies where the problem lies, and the issues faced by civil society.

Let us take a look at the situation surrounding the injunctions filed against nuclear power plants. Residents of Shiga have filed an injunction against the restart of Tsuruga Nuclear Power Plant, arguing that an accident there would contaminate Lake Biwa and threaten the lives of all residents in the Kinki region. In Kyushu, an additional injunction has been filed opposing the operation of all reactors at Genkai Nuclear Power Plant in Saga Prefecture. The issue will continue to become more important as lawsuits opposing nuclear power are filed throughout the country.

Each case was considered separately in the past, but in response to the accident in Fukushima, people have begun to cooperate on a nation-wide scale in the form of anti-nuclear legal teams. These movements can be understood as being aimed at building a society that doesn't depend on nuclear power. In that regard, their movement can be linked to the issues surrounding compensation claims for damage caused by nuclear accidents and disasters.

IV. Conclusion

As previously mentioned, the process for claiming damage compensation has already begun, and collective applications have begun to be considered by the nuclear power ADR organization. However, the situation is still fluid, and the possibility of drastic changes being made to the framework surrounding the damage compensation process itself cannot be ruled out.

It is anticipated that there will be many hurdles to overcome in resolving the issues, and it will take much time. There are many unsolved issues remaining, and it is necessary to observe future trends with calm consideration. To that end, we should consider what sort of society produces a technology that is essentially uncontrollable, and what sort of recovery can be achieved when that technology wipes out the foundation upon which our lives are built.

Acknowledgments

I would like to express my gratitude in writing to the many lawyers whose informative opinions aided me greatly in the writing of this article. They include the legal experts and other individuals from the bar associations and victim legal counsel teams who provided victim consultation support in Saitama and took part in the Disaster Countermeasure Liaison Committee. I also received many excellent suggestions during the JSA-sponsored nuclear disaster lecture series and subsequent discussions. I would like to pass on my heartfelt thanks to all those connected to the legal organizations involved in its operation.

References

Shimizu, S., 2011. *Genpatsu ni nao chiiki no mirai wo takuseru ka.* [Can we still trust the future of our rural areas to nuclear power?], Jichitai Kenkyūsha.

Tokushu 2 - Higashi nihon daishinsai to genpatsu jiko, pāto 2. [Feature 2 - Great East Japan earthquake and nuclear power plant accident, Series 2.], 2011. *Kankyō to Kōgai* (Research on Environmental Disruption), 41 (2), Iwanami Shoten.

Tokushu 3.11 Daishinsai no kōhōgaku, pāto 2. [Feature - Public law regarding the 11 May Earthquake, Part 2.], 2011. *Hōgaku Seminā* [Legal Seminar], 56 (12), 683, Nippon Hyōronsha.

AFTERWORD

The Potential and the Future of Human Sciences
Contributing to Disaster Recovery

Hiroaki Kumano MD, PhD [1][2][3] *(Psychosomatic and Behavioral Medicine)*

Key words: historic disaster, awakening, role of human sciences

On March 11, 2011, the Japanese people faced the greatest disaster in the nation's memory when an earthquake struck off the coast of Fukushima Prefecture in northeastern Japan. That event is now known as the Great East Japan Earthquake Disaster, or more simply as the 2011 Tohoku earthquake, after the Japanese name for the region. This publication brings together the records of the educators and researchers of the Faculty of Human Sciences at Waseda University in their continued efforts to help the region rebuild.

The 2011 Tohoku earthquake was the catalyst for a great awakening among the people of Japan, who, 70 years after the end of the Second World War, had come to view "peace" as the norm. First, it sparked off political and social movements required to overcome the national crisis, and to a greater or lesser extent, all citizens found in that tragedy the motivation to take the first step towards living a life of greater awareness. Waseda University's Faculty of Human Sciences, alongside its affiliated Advanced Research Center for Human Sciences, aims to "solve the problems of humanity". The circumstances surrounding the earthquake led the members of both institutions to resolve to do all they could to help rebuild the country, and the individual who has played the central role in these efforts is Takuya Tsujiuchi, supervising editor of this book and professor at the Faculty of Human Sciences.

---

[1] Director, Advanced Research Center for Human Sciences, Waseda University
[2] Professor, Faculty of Human Sciences, Waseda University
[3] Waseda Institute of Medical Anthropology on Disaster Reconstruction (WIMA)

Professor Tsujiuchi conducted work in the disaster area, but began to consider what he and his colleagues could offer that no one else could. That led to the building of a collaborative relationship with the Shinsai Shien (Earthquake Disaster Support) Network Saitama to help people who had evacuated from Fukushima Prefecture to Saitama, where our faculty is located. It was also the beginning of our efforts to conduct interview surveys in various forms and to provide a multi-faceted support framework based in the data gathered there. However, through that process, Professor Tsujiuchi realized that in order to become a more substantial part of recovery efforts we needed the knowledge and skills of experts, so he visited the US to study with the Harvard Program in Refugee Trauma at Harvard University's School of Public Health. On his return to Japan, he established the Waseda Institute of Medical Anthropology on Disaster Reconstruction, and since then, he has continued to conduct his work as the institute's director.

Bringing the institute's members together, Professor Tsujiuchi was able to acquire the competitive funding offered by the Advanced Research Center for Human Sciences to conduct his research into the human science of reconstruction, and the publication of this book is yet another achievement.

Part I provides a concrete look into the fieldwork and practical efforts the Tsujiuchi laboratory conducted in collaboration with the Shinsai Shien Network, to provide evacuees with the support they needed during the emergency evacuation phase and afterwards, when disaster victims were settling into life as evacuees. Part II brings together a vast array of research conducted by members of the laboratory, made up of educators in the Faculty of Human Sciences teaching a diverse array of specialties, and in particular, visiting researchers who collaborated with us and provided guidance in multiple ways.

Our hope is that you will carefully read about the research conducted by the individual team members, but it is worth noting that the diverse range of research projects included within this book were conducted simultaneously, and through that experience in research, practical implementation and education, we at the faculty have taken a major step forward in the development of Human Science as a discipline. It was a valuable experience which, when the Human Sciences aim to resolves issues as historic as these, the discipline can be best summarized as an "academic integration of practical sciences." This is also reflected in Professor Tsujiuchi's written statement on the purpose of the project, namely, "The Tohoku earthquake was an event of historic proportions, and the Human Sciences were born the moment we took up the shared objective of conducting research that would help the disaster area, as a truly academically integrated and practical discipline able to overcome the multiple issues requiring different types of expertise." I am convinced that Human Sciences will contribute more and more to disaster reconstruction in the future by returning the results of our research to the disaster areas, which will result in the further enhancement of practical implementations.

This book is the culmination of the continuous efforts to help rebuild the Tohoku region made by the many researchers and practitioners connected to the Faculty of Human Sciences at Waseda University. However, it is of the utmost importance that the Japanese people never forget this event, and in view of that, this book can be considered no more than a milestone on our journey to rebuild Japanese society as a whole. We at the Waseda University's Faculty of Human Sciences and Advanced Research Center for Human Sciences aim to grow as individuals as we contribute wholeheartedly to the reconstruction and continued evolution of Japanese society, by gaining an ever-broadening perspective and working to resolve the issues facing humanity with ever-increasing awareness.